Taming the Anxious Mind

A GUIDE BOOK TO RELIEVE STRESS AND ANXIETY

Heidi Schreiber-Pan, Ph.D.

First Printing: 2019

ISBN 978-1-7329988-0-3

Chesapeake Publication
1010 Dulaney Valley Road
Towson, MD 21013

www.chesapeakepublication.com
www.heidischreiberpan.com

Edited by Jeff Karon
Cover design by Lizaa
Illustrations by Sebastian Schreiber-Pan
Typesetting by Sebastian Schreiber-Pan

Printed in the United States of America

Dedication

This book is dedicated to all who struggle with stress and anxiety, and who need support on their journey to finding peace.

To my children, Sebastian and Payton. To my family in Germany, especially my parents, Carol and Kurt and sister, Petra.

Gratitude

To all my professors, mentors and colleagues. My clients, who have taught me so much. Phil Hosmer, writer and friend, who has provided me with valuable feedback from the start. Sebastian, my son and artist who made this book aesthetically pleasing. Lastly, to my husband and partner in all things, Morrison – thank you for your encouragement, unflagging support and love.

Dr. Heidi Schreiber-Pan deconstructs anxiety with narratives and metaphors. She introduces readers to practical tools to help manage stress. She is transparent in her own struggle with anxiety and offers relatable exercises and visual representations. A delightful read and pragmatic guide. Taming the Anxious Mind is a must have for every clinician's bookshelf!

Cheryl Fisher, Ph.D., author, Mindfulness and Nature-Based Interventions for Kids

Life's current frantic pace and the pressure to keep up with technology, new ideas, and life's on-going demands saturate our lives with stress and frustration. Dr. Heidi Schreiber-Pan guides us through a remarkably effective antidote that can help us regain our emotional and psychological balance by reviewing our priorities and gaining back control of our thoughts, feelings, and behaviors and by utilizing a road map that enables us to nurture the most important relationship we have – our self.

Sharon Cheston, Ed.D., author, *Faded Rainbows: Psychospiritual Therapeutic Journeys*

Dr. Heidi Schreiber-Pan's book provides real life examples about issues that make us feel stressed out and anxious, and the tools to help us learn to deal with our stressors and manage our anxiety in healthy ways. Dr. Schreiber-Pan's book includes exercises that involve writing techniques with well-established effectiveness in helping to reduce feelings of anxiety in both Clinical and Counseling Psychology fields. This book is a truly valuable book for those who want to learn how to help themselves.

Kim Shifren, Ph.D., author, *How Caregiving Affects Development: Psychological Implications for Child, Adolescent, and Adult caregivers.*

If I were looking for a therapist to help me meet my anxiety wisely and compassionately, I would hope that I wandered into Heidi Schreiber-Pan's office! This book is a treasure chest filled with well-tested ways to hold a worrying mind and a constricted body in a larger space of kind awareness. You will find help within.

Gordon Peerman, author, *Blessed Relief: What Christians Can Learn from Buddhists about Suffering.*

This book is an easy, clear, and personable support tool for persons who are in therapy and for persons who are ambivalent or not interested in therapy. Dr. Schreiber-Pan uses positive psychology, mindfulness, spirituality and faith integration, and clinical illustrations for readers to recognize that they are not alone struggling with anxiety. Each chapter provides words of wisdom and practical practice exercises for self-empowerment. This book is a must-read for mental health professionals and for every human being who will experience anxiety and stress-related experiences.

Rev. C. Kevin Gillespie, S.J., Ph.D., Psychologist of Religion, Pastor Holy Trinity Church, Washington DC

Taming the Anxious Mind, replete with easy-to-follow exercises and tangible examples, functions as an owner's manual for one's mind.

Phil Hosmer, President, Nature Worx Inc.

Table of Contents

Introduction

One evening, an elderly Cherokee brave told his grandson about a battle that goes on inside people. He said, "My son, the battle is between two 'wolves' inside us all. One is evil. It is anger, envy, jealousy, sorrow, regret, greed, arrogance, self-pity, guilt, resentment, inferiority, lies, false pride, superiority, and ego. The other is good. It is joy, peace, love, hope, serenity, humility, kindness, benevolence, empathy, generosity, truth, compassion, and faith." The grandson thought about it for a minute and then asked his grandfather, "Which wolf wins?" The old Cherokee simply replied, "The one that you feed."

Feeding the Good Wolf

A few summers' ago, my family and I made a trip to the Pacific Northwest, in particular, Vancouver Island, a most magnificent place with its lush green mountains towering out of secluded pockets of freshwater lakes, a place where bald eagles fly freely among the treetops of ancient hemlocks. There we entered the temperate rainforest trail.

A forest of trees so huge, tall and ancient we all looked like little children beside them. A world of vivid green moss, arching ferns, and a mass of plants so thick it's impossible to see the soil beneath them. This trail graced us with an abundance of green in more shades than one can count. The sacredness of this place struck us almost immediately. All talk ceased with the overwhelming need to take in this sensual experience. It was like a rare glimpse into the beginning of Creation: fresh, pristine, untouched, sanctified. I could feel the presence of nature in every fiber of my being. This moment of awe in nature was creating peace, joy and excitement—in other words, this experience was feeding the good wolf within me. My hope is that the teachings, stories, metaphors, illustrations, practices and reflections offered in this book help you nourish the good wolf within yourself so that wolf can become the dominant animal, the alpha of your life.

My Own Dance with Anxiety

When my son, Sebastian, was ten years old, he contracted MRSA, a difficult to treat bacterial infection. The first sign of the sickness was a painful, swollen, red area on his lower back.

Once the fever set in, we rushed him off to the doctors. After several tests, we were told about MRSA. That summer, a teenager from our community had died of the same disease. My anxiety spiraled out of control. I was in full-blown fight or flight response. Not eating, not sleeping, with imagery of worse-case scenarios running through my head. I could not handle losing my child. As the medication finally cleared up the infection, the relief that washed over me was of epic proportions. I began sobbing; with each forceful exhalation, the anxiety subsided. That event initiated a lifelong dance with anxiety. At times, anxiety flares up and wants to take control of my days. However, I have acquired the skill of leading this dance. Managing my anxiety is similar to the line shared by Jon Kabat-Zinn: "You can't stop the waves, but you can learn to surf." Taming the Anxious Mind will equip you with ways to lead your own dance with anxiety.

Building a Healthy Relationship with the Mind

My role as a therapist includes coaching people on their relationship with the mind. Think about it. When did you learn about the functions or nature of the mind? Chances are you never really learned about it. And yet the mind supervises all your experiences. The mind can be understood as a system that runs complex cognitive processes such as thinking and feeling.

Most of us have a peculiar relationship with the mind, which can be summed up as the mind being the master and you being the servant. Riding a horse that is untrained leaves us at the mercy of its every whim. If the horse wants to eat grass, we are left standing there. If the horse decides to run, we are thrown wildly about. So, it is with a mind that is left untrained. If the mind wants to spout negative ideas, we are left feeling miserable. If the mind decides to imagine worse-case-scenarios, we experience intense anxiety. *Taming the Anxious Mind* is a quick-guide to building a sustainable and healthy relationship with your mind.

A Unique Recipe

As a psychotherapist, I'm constantly on the lookout for ways to transform constructs of harm into hands-on, applicable practices that are easy to integrate into daily life yet have immense positive effects. This user-friendly book offers a unique therapeutic recipe to help tackle your personal experience of anxiety and stress. From doing therapy for over twenty years, attending neuroscientific trainings, teaching college students, conducting research and personal experiences, I have collected valuable data that highlights human resiliency. This recipe is an invitation for you to become the architect of your own happiness.

Taming the Anxious Mind is not meant to be simply read or skimmed over in front of the fireplace with a cup of herbal tea steaming next to you. The content of each chapter is meant for you to absorb and, most importantly, practice.

My own professional path of speaking to diverse audiences has taught me that people can connect with stories and metaphors on a very deep level. Foundational stories of various wisdom and faith traditions invite us to make meaning of our own experiences of joy and suffering. Therefore, each chapter invites the reader on a journey of uncovering the story's personal relevance before diving into the informative portion of the material. Finally, it is critical to create time and space to engage with the end-of-chapter practices. Let's take to heart the words of Benjamin Franklin:

> *"Tell me and I forget, teach me and I may remember, involve me and I learn."*

1

I Am Stressed

A psychologist walked around a room while teaching stress management to an audience. As she raised a glass of water, everyone expected they'd be asked the "half empty or half full" question. Instead, with a smile on her face, she inquired, "How heavy is this glass of water?" Answers called out ranged from 8 oz. to 20 oz.

She replied, "The absolute weight doesn't matter. It depends on how long I hold it. If I hold it for a minute, it's not a problem. If I hold it for an hour, I'll have an ache in my arm. If I hold it for a day, my arm will feel numb and paralyzed. In each case, the weight of the glass doesn't change, but the longer I hold it, the heavier it becomes." She continued, "The stresses and worries in life are like that glass of water. Think about them for a while and nothing happens. Think about them a bit longer and they begin to hurt. And if you think about them all day long, you will feel paralyzed—incapable of doing anything."

It's important to remember to let go of your stresses. As early in the evening as you can, put all your burdens down. Don't carry them through the evening and into the night. Remember to put the glass down!

I Am Stressed

Think, for a minute, about what causes stress in your life. Perhaps you juggle a lot of roles and responsibilities. Maybe you are trying to figure out how to pick up the children from school as the conference call is running late while the new puppy is ready for potty break number three. Perhaps you are feeling stressed because you are working as hard as you can, and your income is still insufficient in meeting all your financial obligations—college tuition is an outrage these days! Maybe you are newly retired and have lots of free time, but the lack of meaning and purpose is creating a sense of unease and restlessness.

We all carry our share of burdens. Burdens aren't harmful as long as we can remember "to put it down" as instructed by the psychologist and that glass of water. This book is about how to put down your glass of stress on a regular basis in order to successfully manage anxiety, worry and disease.

The Stress Wave Is Coming

Imagine transforming all your stressors into the image of a wave. Come on: Give your imagination free range and envision an ocean wave filled with all the things in your life that are currently creating stress. Is your wave small and brief, more like a ripple? For some people, their wave feels like a tsunami or tidal wave. Now imagine swimming a few feet from shore, floating peacefully on the beautiful ocean water, when a large wave is heading directly towards you.

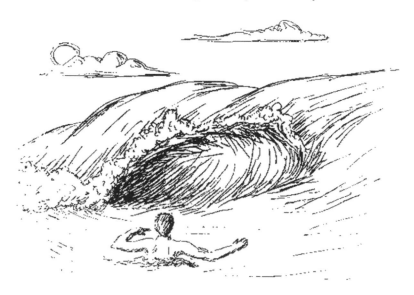

What are your options? You can either dive under the wave, you can try to ride the wave out to the shore or you can let the swell crash into your body. We will explore the first two options in hopes that you can learn to avoid the crash.

Diving Under

When we choose to dive under the wave, we immediately encounter a brief moment of stillness as the water tumbles above our heads onto the shore. If you ever experienced scuba diving or even snorkeling, you noticed that under the surface of the water lies calm and stillness, a quiet landscape teeming with life. I am here to tell you that this same stillness is within all of us: We simply need to learn the skill to reach it. One way to uncover this stillness is to remain anchored in the present moment.

Why is it so difficult to remain in the here and now? Our minds are bound to contemplate past events or anticipate future happenings. Anxiety thrives when we exert our mental energy on future-oriented thought processes such as the never ending "what if's," to-do lists and ought-to's. It's been said that Mark Twain as well as Winston Churchill once remarked that their lives were filled with many terrible misfortunes, most of which never happened. Our mind has the most powerful capacity to create elaborate fictions in which we play out every aspect of the "worst case scenario." Understandably, such fictions will incite intense anxiety. Our mind is quite content ruminating and chewing on past situations, particularly the ones that were upsetting in some way. Often people who suffer from depression spend an enormous amount of mental resources rehashing past events. An intentional practice of anchoring oneself in the present moment has the power to create freedom from the entrapping influence of the past and future.

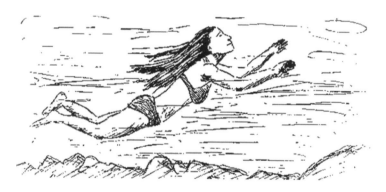

One helpful way to observe present-moment-living is through both a formal and informal practice of mindfulness. Mindfulness can be understood as the practice of anchoring or tuning into what is going on at this very moment. The magic happens the instant we recognize that we are cruising on autopilot and then deliberately disengage from the mind machine. A formal practice could incorporate a 10-minute guided mindfulness meditation exercise, to help you check in with your body, where you receive instructions to mentally scan down your body from head to toe. An informal practice can include becoming aware and paying attention to mundane daily tasks such as eating, showering or doing the dishes—not simply mindlessly taking a shower but consciously paying attention to the aroma of the soap and feeling of the water on the skin. Future chapters will discuss these practices in more detail.

Ride the Wave

When the timing is just right, and the body is perfectly positioned, it can be exhilarating to ride an ocean wave all the way out onto the shore. More often than not, the timing or body position is a bit off, and one experiences the rough tumble of the surf. Sometimes that means a few scratches and scrapes, burning from the saltwater. Certain life storms and crises are going to throw us to the ground in such a violent matter that all we can do is bear our suffering, one deep breath at a time. We don't have the time or wherewithal to dive under the surface. When a loved one dies, when we lose our job, when our spouse is having an affair, or when our child is diagnosed with cancer, we must bear witness to our storm as we batten down the hatches, trusting that this storm will pass.

Not even hurricanes last forever! This is a time when conscious breathing can carry us from one hour to the next, where love and support from family and friends are indispensable tools that guarantee our survival for yet one more day.

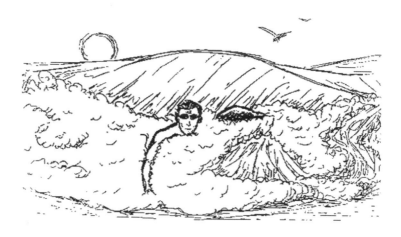

The Case of Emily

Some years ago, a young woman enrolled in a stress reduction course that I offered. Emily had recently given birth to a little girl and encountered unexpected hardship in her role as a new mother. Her baby was often cranky, repeatedly sick with the common cold, awake long into the night, and her husband turned out to be little help. Emily found herself submerged in negativity. She described her wave as crushing, forceful and relentless. In class, she shared an instance in which her baby woke up at 2 am, shortly after Emily had finally fallen asleep. Emily was completely miserable as she held her daughter in her arms. Nothing was going right—wasn't motherhood supposed to be wonderful?

There is nothing wonderful about being sleep-deprived in addition to being assaulted by the wailing of an infant. The moment of riding the wave had arrived. However, Emily wasn't riding the wave: She was fighting it. She was stiffly standing her ground while the wave crashed into her body. Buddhist philosophy tells us that pain is inevitable, but suffering is optional. In Emily's case, she added suffering to this unavoidable situation through letting her thoughts spin a toxic web, thoughts such as *"This situation is unbearable," "Something is wrong," "I hate my husband for sleeping right now," "I am not a good mother," "I won't function tomorrow with such little sleep."* Throughout the following weeks, Emily began a formal 10-minute mindfulness practice along with monitoring her negative, unhelpful thoughts.

Her baby still wakes her up in the middle of the night. Now Emily is better equipped to ride the wave: one breath at a time, bearing witness to her discomfort and sleepiness without adding negative thought processes to magnify her distress. In some way, Emily is letting go of thoughts and stories about what "should be" happening and is saying "yes" to what is happening in that moment. Buddhist principles affirm the notion that resistance to one's current experience is at the heart of suffering. What one resists persists. However, an attitude of acceptance can dissipate uncomfortable feelings. Motherhood includes moments of wonder and awe as well as moments of frustration and misery; all feelings have a place at the table. All need to be welcomed.

Practice: Stressor Write-Off

----

1. Make a list of all the current stressors in your life that cause anxiety, worry, pressure or strain. The list can include situations, people, fears or thoughts.

2. Convert all the stressors into the image of a wave. Draw your wave. Describe your wave.

3. Notice how writing about stressors often brings a sense of relief. Something therapeutic happens when we can externalize our troubles. Consequently, many psychological studies describe the positive effect of journaling on psychological well-being as writing literally helps "get it off your chest." Create a habit of recording thoughts on paper. Experience the relief of discharging your cares. This is especially helpful when a noisy mind is keeping you from falling asleep at night.

Practice: Reflective Writing Exercise

----

1. Look at the Words of Wisdom page of quotes. Choose a quote that speaks to you. Why is this quote meaningful to you? In what way do you have need for that wisdom in your life?

2. What thoughts and feelings bubble up for you when you look at the wave image and your list of stressors?

3. What keeps you from experiencing that peace that is available "below the surface"?

4. What role does your faith or spirituality play when struggling with difficulties?

Words of Wisdom

- *"Feelings come and go like clouds in a windy sky. Conscious breathing is my anchor."* Thich Nhat Hanh

- *"The greatest weapon against stress is our ability to choose one thought over another."* William James

- *"The word worry is derived from an old Anglo-Saxon word meaning to 'strangle or choke.' The stranglehold of worry keeps a woman from enjoying a life of contentment and peace."* Linda Dillow

- *"The fears that assault us are mostly simple anxieties about social skills, about intimacy, about likeableness, or about performance. We need not give emotional food or charge to these fears or become attached to them. We don't even have to shame ourselves for having these fears. Simply ask your fears, 'What are you trying to teach me?' Some say that FEAR is merely an acronym for 'False Evidence Appearing Real.'"* Richard Rohr

- *When we are in the midst of chaos, let go of the need to control it. Be awash in it, experience it in that moment, try not to control the outcome but deal with the flow as it comes."* Leo Babauta

- *"Notice that the stiffest tree is the most easily cracked, while the bamboo or willow survives by bending with the wind."* Bruce Lee

- *"The secret of health for both mind and body is not to mourn for the past, not to worry about the future, not to anticipate the future, but to live the present moment wisely and earnestly."* Buddha

- *"We don't realize that, somewhere within us all, there does exist a supreme self who is eternally at peace."* Elizabeth Gilbert

29

2   Why Am I So Anxious?

"Once there was a young warrior. Her teacher told her that she had to do battle with fear. She didn't want to do that. It seemed too aggressive; it was scary; it seemed unfriendly. But the teacher said she had to do it and gave her the instructions for the battle. The day arrived. The student warrior stood on one side, and fear stood on the other. The warrior was feeling very small, and fear was looking big and wrathful. They both had their weapons. The young warrior roused herself and went toward fear, prostrated three times, and asked, 'May I have permission to go into battle with you?' Fear said, 'Thank you for showing me so much respect that you ask permission.' Then the young warrior said, 'How can I defeat you?' Fear replied, 'My weapons are that

I talk fast, and I get very close to your face. Then you get completely unnerved, and you do whatever I say. If you don't do what I tell you, I have no power. You can listen to me, and you can have respect for me. You can even be convinced by me. But if you don't do what I say, I have no power.' In that way, the student warrior learned how to defeat fear."

(Pema Chödrön, When Things Fall Apart: Heart Advice for Difficult Times)

Why so Anxious

Once upon a time, through the complex process of evolution, human beings developed into highly functioning and thriving individuals and operational societies. Thanks to our survival instinct, people learned to effectively scan the environment for threats to their safety. Our ancestors would constantly check their surroundings for dangers or problems to fix. Back then, it was a matter of life and death to detect a bear lurking in the shadows or to find a solution to ineffective food storage systems. Consequently, our brains developed a negativity bias, habitually seeking out negative stimuli. Such primitive responses have accompanied us to the present day and often do much harm.

The anxiety response has been millions of years in the making. Today, it is not the bear that threatens our survival but our brain's interpretation of being stuck in traffic, family conflict or looming deadlines. Our brain does not have the ability to comprehend that being late to an interview isn't actually life-threatening. This false perception gives rise to the automatic fight or flight response that often includes dizziness, heart pounding, tension, jaw clenching, dry mouth, gastrointestinal issues, tightness in the throat and chest or difficulty breathing. A prolonged or chronic experience of the fight or flight reaction can have serious health and mental health consequences. Our bodies simply cannot sustain this tension long-term. Therefore, it is essential to learn ways of engaging the body's natural relaxation response, which originates in our body's parasympathetic nervous system.

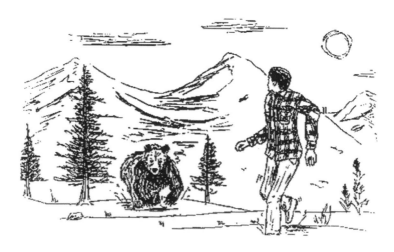

When we perceive a real threat, our body activates the fight or flight response. Consequently, the body begins a process of intensification with the sole intention of protecting the body. Our sympathetic nervous system directs all resources toward fighting off a threat or fleeing from danger. Anxiety or worry is caused by experiencing many fearful thoughts which in turn activate this biological alarm system. Without realizing it, one develops a pattern of responding to situations in a fearful manner, consequently activating fight or flight inappropriately. If this pattern persists long enough, one feels constantly on edge and begins to believe that this feeling is normal, convincing oneself "that's just how I am."

Fear vs. Anxiety

The experience of anxiety is often a misinterpretation of a harmless stimulus as a dangerous threat. It's not the act of dropping the children off late to school that is causing the clenching of the jaw but the belief that the delayed arrival at school is a sure sign of our inability to be a responsible parent.

Evolutionary theory tells us that our body has an innate drive to ensure our survival through consistent attention to possible hazards coming our way. For example, if one encounters a bear in the wild, the fight or flight response is activated immediately. Anxiety, on the other hand, is oriented to the future and the possibility of seeing a bear. Fear is associated with a clear and present danger. Anxiety can occur in the absence of actual danger.

- o Fear: seeing a bear vs. Anxiety: the possibility of seeing a bear
- o Fear: being fired from your job vs. Anxiety: the possibility of being fired from your job
- o Fear: being robbed vs. Anxiety: the chance of being robbed
- o Fear: suffering an injury vs. Anxiety: the chance of being injured

The mind is very crafty at convincing you that a bear will attack you while hiking a trail even though it's only a very slight possibility. After all, the mind's opinion feels like truth——it's right there inside of your head. However, the mind's opinions are simply a collection of thoughts, not indisputable facts. The student warrior was able to reject such opinions, hence stand victorious in the end.

The Case of Olivia

Balancing an active home life with her part-time career as a classical musician was becoming an increasingly difficult assignment. Moreover, Olivia was spending time she did not have on compulsive rituals such as checking the stove and her curling iron. Her toddler would curiously watch as she consistently drove back up the driveway to perform her "just making sure" habits. Her mind would create persistent thinking patterns that assured her of the impending danger of a plugged-in curling iron, even though she was sure she had unplugged it prior to exiting her bathroom. However, the mind would generate numerous doubts, forcing her to return to the house after she barely even left her neighborhood.

Anxiety feeds on negative emotions and thoughts, consequently activating the fight or flight response, often with a chronic frequency. For instance, anxiety will initiate thoughts such as these:

> *"Do you remember the story on the news about the house that burned down? If you left that curling iron on, the house will catch fire. You must go back and check; otherwise, it will be all your fault."*

In time, Olivia learned to engage her thinking mind rather than simply believe it. "Yes, it is possible that I left the curling iron on. However, it is highly unlikely that the house would burn down. Of course, I would not want our house to burn down, but I cannot control everything in life. However, I need to work with my anxiety, and so I'm going to take the risk that I left the iron plugged in and keep driving anyway without going back to check. I believe in my ability to handle this." Olivia, being a devout Catholic, chose to end her mantra with Philippians 4:13: *"I can do all things through Christ who strengthens me."* She continued saying her script until her anxiety slowly decreased and she was well on her way down the road.

Practice: Getting to Know My Anxiety

When you think about your relationship with your anxiety, you may use words to describe it such as tense, frustrating or afraid. Here is an invitation to change your relationship with anxiety by simply becoming more curious about it. These questions may help you investigate your experience of anxiety from a curious and less judgmental viewpoint.

1. What are some common triggers that elicit anxiety in you? Common triggers include family conflict, perfectionism, work pressures, unmet expectations, overloaded schedule, etc.

2. Try to verbalize the thoughts you have when experiencing anxiety?

3. How do you typically respond to anxiety? In other words, what coping mechanism do you use? These can be healthy ways of coping (e.g., exercising, counseling, calling a friend) or unhealthy ways of coping (e.g., drinking, withdrawing, being irritable).

Practice: Where in My Body

Become curious about the sensations in your body as you experience anxiety. In the picture below, indicate where in the body you feel any anxiety symptoms. Be precise, describe the sensation in detail.

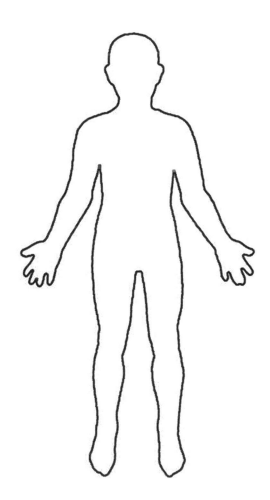

3 Anxiety—My Unwanted Family Member

On a beautiful summer day, my family set out to hike part of the Appalachian Trail through Great Smoky Mountains National Park. The trail was very well maintained overall. However, a small section of the trail went through a thicket and forest undergrowth. I was unaware of the dangers lurking in the fauna: poison ivy. A few days later, my legs showed the all-too-familiar nasty, red, blistering rash. Anyone who has experienced this wicked form of torture knows about the intense urge to scratch the irritation. I gave in to the itch and consequently made things worse: the rash spread all over my body. Scratching brought about a brief sense of relief yet did not help alleviate the inflammation. My body needed me to stop scratching and allow for healing to begin.

Similarly, the anxiety itch urges you to find some way to relieve your body and mind from the discomfort of feeling fearful. When it comes to anxiety, avoidance equals relief. So, you begin avoiding whatever triggers your anxiety: social situations, flying, dating, interviewing, etc. Avoidance, however, makes things worse. It fuels the anxiety, making it bigger and stronger.

Now it may be easier to avoid poison ivy than things that trigger your anxiety. However, when you scratch your anxiety itch, it makes the anxiety worse and can eventually spread to infect your whole life.

My Anxious Side

Recently, I discovered that I am not quite as extroverted as I used to think. I enjoy being with people, but if I am honest, extended time with people can deplete my energy. Thus, time to myself often feels like a replenishing of much needed life-power. Consequently, I have come to honor my introverted side through careful inclusion of "silence and solitude" into my schedule. There is room for various aspects of my personality: the extroverted, socially-engaged me and the introverted, quiet solitary me. Respecting the needs of both sides has created a more balanced lifestyle.

What if some people have an anxious component of self, in other words, an anxious side to one's experience of self? Would it make sense to avoid or get rid of a part of ourselves? Healthy living necessitates acceptance of every ingredient that makes up who we are, including our undesirable parts. Will you allow room for the anxious, angry or sad side of your existence?

The attitude of allowing emotions to flow through our experience is a direct antidote to habitually reacting to strong emotions such as scratching an anxiety itch.

Chinese Finger Trap

This small bamboo cylinder has been used for ages to play practical jokes on unsuspecting victims whose fingers get trapped inside the toy once people try to pull their fingers out of the cylinder. What people often fail to notice is that the very movement of pushing the fingers deeper inside the trap causes the bamboo to loosen and consequently frees the fingers by creating more space and wiggle room.

The anxiety trap is surprisingly similar. One spends an incredible amount of energy trying to get out of experiencing anxiety, yet the more one tries to get rid of it, the more persistent anxiety becomes. Our instincts are convincingly strong, and often it feels like we have no choice but to pull away.

The alternative approach goes against the grain. It suggests pushing in instead of pulling out. Giving in, or acceptance, generates more space, more wiggle room. As you allow the discomfort of the emotion to exist, you are pushing in and making room for all the different parts of you.

Tip: Positive self-talk can be highly effective in reducing the intensity of anxiety and depression. *"My anxiety is making me feel uncomfortable, yet I allow the discomfort to be here. I allow it to be here and won't try to make it go away."*

Anxiety is like a Chinese Finger Trap. The more you struggle with things you're afraid of, the more imprisoned you become.

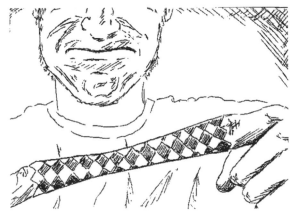

Don't Believe Everything You Think

"Cogito ergo sum," translated as the famous Descartes quote "I think; therefore, I am," points to the philosophical notion of the entanglement of thought and existence. Some people erroneously interpret this idea as proof that our thoughts make up who we are. In other words, the voice we hear in our mind embodies our soul, our self.

I have come to accept an opposing notion. Thoughts are merely brain processes without any reliable connection to reality. This notion is life-giving, liberating and can be a tremendously helpful when working with stress or anxiety. For example, if you are aware of the thought "I can't handle this" and you assure yourself that this thought is not a fact, but a mere brain process triggered by feeling overwhelmed, you can begin working with the mind instead of accepting this unhelpful thought as truth. What I mean by "working" with the mind is the act of witnessing the thoughts as they move through one's awareness, not unlike the news ticker that propels various stories along at the bottom of people's TV screens. It's been said that nearly 80% of human thought processes contain negative matter. That in itself isn't inherently problematic. However, the human impulse to believe those thoughts can lead to disaster. A natural antidote to this impulse is to step back and ask oneself, "Is this thought true?" "How is believing this thought making me feel right now?"

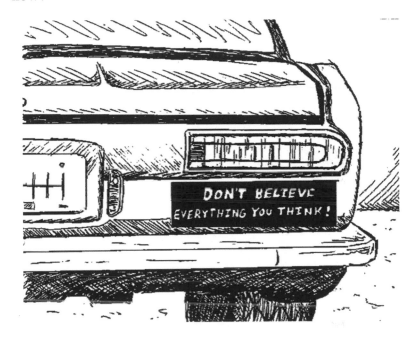

Our Relationship with Anxiety: The Unwanted Family Member

Remember the Chinese finger trap analogy? I would like to offer another allegory that may be helpful in evolving one's relationship with anxiety from one loaded with resistance to one approaching acceptance. Imagine that you are preparing to host Thanksgiving dinner. You don't particularly enjoy your cousin Oscar who is quite obnoxious and often makes you feel uncomfortable with his larger-than-life personality. However, he is part of the family and has a right to be there just as every other member of the family. You remind yourself that you only need to endure him for a few hours before you return to your peaceful post-holiday life (yeah right!). What if you could have that kind of relationship with your anxiety? What if anxiety is part of your experience just as happiness is a part? In some way, welcoming anxiety to the Thanksgiving table, knowing that it has a right to be there and that it will eventually leave again, can reduce the intensity of that emotion.

The Case of Dan

Recently, I worked with a middle-aged man who had lost his job with a well-paying construction company. He was very distraught over the loss of his job and wanted help examining the events that led up to his discharge. Dan had a history of mild anxiety, particularly during high-stress times at work. One day, he was driving to the location of the next job which involved crossing the Chesapeake Bay Bridge, a large suspension span rising to 186 feet above the water. After paying the toll, he simultaneously noticed several things happening in his body. Dan's heart was pounding, the chest and throat area felt constricted, and it was difficult to breathe.

Dan rushed to alleviate his discomfort. As soon as he turned around and headed away from the bridge, his anxiety decreased until…Dan arrived at the Delaware Memorial Bridge (175 feet above the water) and entered into panic again. As he continued avoiding bridges, small and large, he often ran late to jobs and was ultimately laid off.

Replaying the memory of the Bay Bridge event during sessions, Dan became aware of how he had scratched his anxiety itch. First, he fueled the fire of his anxiety by allowing himself to think more and more fearful thoughts such as *"It's easy to have an accident on the bridge;" "If I get hit by another car," "I will tumble down the bridge—what a horrible way to die;" "There hasn't been an accident on this bridge for a while, it's overdue;"* and *"Terrorists could easy target this bridge."* Dan's avoidance of driving over the Bay Bridge caused the anxiety to grow and spread. Avoidance as a coping mechanism has a tendency to "infect" other situations and generate more anxiety triggers. Hence, Dan's anxiety about the Bay Bridge spread to other bridges, even relatively low and short structures.

In treatment, Dan learned that the first step out of the vicious anxiety-avoidance cycle was the simple realization that avoidance does not work; in fact, avoidance had only increased his problems and caused him to lose his job and confidence in himself as a competent human being. Furthermore, he acquired tools to help him soothe and regulate anxious emotions.

In essence, Dan no longer avoids his anxious feelings but allows their presence while using his tools to lessen the intensity.

Practice: Waterfall Visualization

Let's invite your imagination to be part of this exercise. Imagine that you are going for a hike on a hot summer day. The air is fresh, the shades of green are vivid, and the forest trail smells of dried pine needles. As you walk along the trail, you see a brilliant waterfall in front of you. You decide to cool off and walk into the swimming hole near the falls. Your curiosity compels you to experiment with sticking your head right underneath the falls. The water feels heavy on your head; the pressure of the flow almost hurts. As you take a step back, the pressure immediately releases from your head, and you stand behind the waterfall and watch as the water plunges in front of you continuously. Similarly, a stream of thoughts endlessly flows through our minds, yet our ability to step behind the waterfall of our thoughts has the potential to release stress and anxiety as we become observers rather than casualties of the pressure.

Practice this visualization several times a day for a few moments. This training of the mind can facilitate more calmness as you begin creating distance between you and your largely negatively-skewed thought processes

4 I Choose Human Flourishing

One evening, an old Cherokee told his grandson about a battle that goes on inside people. He said, "My son, the battle is between two 'wolves' inside us all. One is Evil. It is anger, envy, jealousy, sorrow, regret, greed, arrogance, self-pity, guilt, resentment, inferiority, lies, false pride, superiority and ego. The other is Good. It is joy, peace, love, hope, serenity, humility, kindness, benevolence, empathy, generosity, truth, compassion and faith." The grandson thought about it for a minute and then asked his grandfather, "Which wolf wins?" The old Cherokee simply replied, "The one you feed."

Every Day We Choose

We must return once more to this native American parable to highlight the potential of all humans to do great evil or to do great good. We have the choice every day to think and behave in a way that either nurtures the part of us that is filled with love and peace or the shadow part that is fed by anger and resentment. If we allow our thinking to ruminate on worst-case scenarios and remain on thoughts such as I have every right to be angry, we inadvertently feed the bad wolf and consequently strengthen this wolf's presence in our lives. If we give in to urges of road rage, impatience with the store clerk or nasty remarks to the telemarketer, we fuel the fire of negative emotions.

Even though emotions can seem powerful beyond control, make no mistake: emotions are inherently related to our thinking processes and therefore are well under our control to influence. Every day these two wolves go into battle inside of us, and every day we choose to feed one of them. It is up to us to which wolf will win.

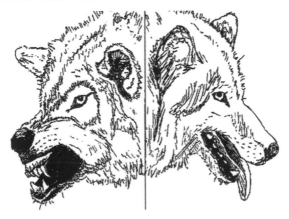

The Positive Psychology of Human Flourishing

What do joy, fun, gratitude, love, peace and happiness have in common? These positive emotions are the cornerstone of the relatively new field of positive psychology. After years of studying psychology in college and memorizing symptomatology, diagnosis criteria and optimal treatment plans, I found it difficult to believe that psychology was anything but a detailed investigation of mental illness and disorder. However, positive psychology's departure from the disease model to focus on human resilience and well-being caused an immediate upheaval in my professional development and future graduate research. Positive psychology is utilized by people who do well even in the face of adversity. This field studies what makes people happy and how to strengthen one's life satisfaction. The very essence of the Declaration of Independence insists that we all hold the right to pursue happiness. The appeal of positive psychology entails the optimistic and encouraging themes of personal growth, self-actualization and human flourishing.

In 2010, Haiti suffered one of the worst natural catastrophes in recent history, a magnitude 7 earthquake. Estimates of human lives lost on that terrible day in January were close to 250,000 people. A few years after the tragedy, I joined a team of researchers from Loyola University, Maryland, to investigate the concept of Post Traumatic Growth (PTG). Unlike its well-known cousin Post Traumatic Stress Disorder (PTSD), PTG looks at the potential for growth after suffering a traumatic event. In the mid-1990s, psychologist Richard Tedeschi, PhD, and Lawrence Calhoun, PhD, developed a theory that speaks of transformation following trauma. In other words, they witnessed that some people who tackled traumatic adversity emerged having personally matured in their understanding of self, others and how to live life.

The findings from the trip and subsequent study suggest that for the highly spiritual or religious people of Haiti, trauma was an impetus for spiritual and personal development and renewal. Survivors' post-trauma functioning seemed to be linked to their interpretations of the events that surrounded the earthquake. Many Haitians found strength and security in the belief that a higher power was present with them during the earthquake. Consequently, Haitians are an extraordinarily resilient folk.

Posttraumatic growth, resilience, psychological well-being and happiness—all of these concepts are studied in the field of positive psychology, and all of these concepts need our individual nourishment for our lives to flourish and thrive, so our good wolf will win.

Emotional Intelligence

Last August, my husband and I dropped our son off at college. In the months leading up to the moment of drop-off, I tried my best to keep it together, pretending that I was totally okay and excited to launch my first born 1,500 miles away from home. My way of dealing with the anticipatory grief was to avoid thinking about it. I didn't even talk to Sebastian about it because I didn't want those sad emotions to show up. I did the very thing that actually created more sadness since "stuffing" emotions are a surefire way of perpetuating emotional pain. Bottling our feelings may seem effortless, but there is an internal consequence which may surface as anger, blame, health problems, anxiety or depression.

Emotional Intelligence (EQ) is the ability to identify and manage your own emotions and the emotions of others. Healthy ways of dealing with emotions can be learned just like any other ability.

Daniel Goleman, a leading expert in the field of emotional intelligence, describes five essential skill-sets evident in highly emotional intelligent individuals. These include self-awareness, self-regulations, motivation, empathy and social skills. Conducting the following internal inquiry can assist you in bringing attention to your EQ abilities:

Self-Awareness

o "What is going on inside of me right now?"

o "What feelings are present in this moment?"

o "Do I trust myself to accomplish what I have set out to do?"

Self-Regulation

o "What can I do to calm myself down when I am upset?"

o "What can I do to cheer myself up when I am feeling down?"

o "What will help me adapt to this new situation?"

Motivation

o "What do I want in life?"

o "Who do I want to be?"

o "What will help me stay committed?"

Empathy

o "What is going on inside this other person right now?"

o "What would it be like to be in his/her place?"

Social Skills

o "How can I communicate in a way that I build bridges and not walls?"

o "What contributions will make me a team player?"

o "How do I become a better listener?"

The Curious Life of a Water Lily

Most of us would agree that the water lily is one of the most breathtaking flowers on Earth. You'd think that a plant of this beauty would grow in some pristine, clear mountain lake. Well, not quite. The water lily flourishes in the muddy, weed-infested waters of dark ponds. Buddhism has pointed to the lily as a metaphor of life: We all encounter mud and darkness on our path, but the ability to turn darkness into beauty is one definition of emotional intelligence.

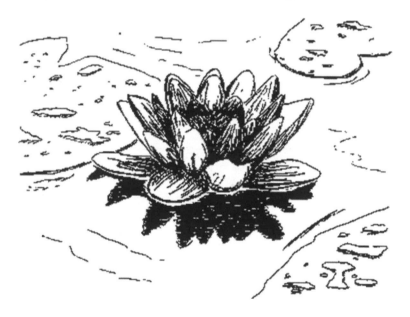

Once we have dwelled on the dark side of an experience, can we encourage ourselves to look at some of the upsides? The "silver lining technique" encourages you to list three positive things about an upsetting situation. For example, you might reflect on how the end of a relationship has given you a chance to now focus on self-care, has allowed you to re-design your life and has created time to rekindle old friendships.

"Whenever you should doubt your self-worth, remember the lotus flower. Even though it plunges to life from beneath the mud, it does not allow the dirt that surrounds it to affect its growth or beauty."

-Suzy Kassem

The Case of Paula

Paula's life was wrought with trauma. At an early age, her father died unexpectedly, leaving her to take care of her younger sister. Her mother was frequently physically as well as emotionally absent due to severe depression. Relatives demanded Paula "man up" now that she was the responsible one (at the ripe age of 10 years old), disapproving of any show of emotions as she grieved the love of her life: her daddy. Paula jumped at the first chance of leaving the family home behind, entering college and soon afterward marrying a classmate. However, the escape turned into years of spousal abuse as her husband often became violent after hours of drinking.

Paula initiated therapy after the death of her spouse. Consumed with resentment and bitterness for a life filled with pain, Paula spent months using therapy to express her anger and brood over the injustice done to her. Paula was feeding the wolf that consumes anger, envy, jealousy, sorrow, regret, self-pity, guilt, resentment, inferiority and lies.

Some Eastern wisdom traditions believe that people can create an internal energy flow that's either positive or negative. This energy has the potential to influence our external environment. In other words, if a person is filled with negative energy, he or she is likely to attract negative life events. Have you ever met a person who seems to have the worst luck?

Along with science, I remain skeptical about this hypothesis. However, in the case of Paula, once she began making intentional changes in her thinking—committing to a daily expressive writing practice, engaging in mindfulness meditation and joining a church community—random acts of "good luck" appeared in her daily life, such as a stranger paying for her lunch at a local fast food place, the car in front of her covering her charge at the toll both, the insurance company paying for a new roof, and a small promotion at work. Is it the metaphysical existence of energy flow or merely her newfound ability to take in the good? Perhaps it doesn't matter as long as we choose to feed the good wolf and are there to witness the benefits.

Practice: Expressive Writing for Rumination

How do you respond when something bad happens? A lot of us relive the event over and over in our minds, recreating the painful moment. Rumination, the act of mulling something over repeatedly, is linked to anxiety and depression. It's like swaying in a rocking chair: It keeps us busy but gets us nowhere.

The practice of expressive writing gives us a chance to change the narrative from predominantly negative forms of rumination to a more meaning-making way of thinking. Many people report that expressive writing has decreased the mind's urge to ruminate. It seems once the thoughts are out on paper, the mind lets go of the need to rehash. Here is how it works:

1) Find a place and time where you are likely to remain uninterrupted.

2) Write for at least 20 minutes (don't stop before 20 minutes is over) about an issue that has brought up difficult emotions.

3) Investigate, then get your deepest thoughts and feelings about the issue out on paper.

4) Let go of grammar and sentence structure—they don't matter!

5) Conclude with the silver lining technique.

My Mind over Matter

Imagine you're given a parrot. This parrot is just a parrot—it doesn't have any knowledge, wisdom or insight. It's bird-brained after all. It recites things "parrot-fashion" without any understanding or comprehension. Like I said, "It's a parrot." However, this particular parrot is a poisoned and poisonous parrot. It's been specifically trained to be unhelpful to you, continuously commenting on you and your life in a way that constantly puts you down, criticizes you.

For example, the bus gets stuck in a traffic jam, and you arrive at work five minutes late. The parrot sits there saying, "There you go again, late. You just can't even manage to get there on time, can you? You're so stupid. If you had left the house and got the earlier bus, you would have arrived with loads of time to spare and the boss would be happy. But you? No way.

Just can't do it. You're a useless waste of space, absolutely pathetic!"

How long would you put up with this abuse before throwing a towel over the cage or getting rid of the parrot? Yet we can often put up with the thoughts from this internal bully for far too long, decades even. We hear that parrot, believe the parrot, and naturally get upset.

That then affects the way we live our lives—the way we behave towards others, how we are, what we think about others, what we think about the world, and how we think and feel about ourselves.

We can learn to use the antidote (or the anti-parrot!): Just notice that parrot and cover the cage! "There's that parrot again. I don't have to listen to it—it's just a parrot," you think.

Then go and do something else. Put your focus of attention on something other than that parrot. This parrot is poison, though, and it won't give up easily, so you'll need to keep using that antidote and be persistent in your practice.

Eventually, it will get tired of the towel, tired of you not responding. You'll notice it less and less. It might just give up its poison as your antidote overcomes it, or perhaps fly off to wherever poisoned parrots go.

Thoughts then Feelings then Behaviors

Sarah, a client I recently began working with, shared this story with me. She had moved into a new neighborhood and was looking forward to meeting new neighbors and making friends. Just a week after she had moved in, someone had told her that the neighborhood was holding a summer happy hour for the community. Sarah was excited to attend but felt nervous showing up at the gathering by herself. Nevertheless, she got herself ready, took heart and walked into the backyard gathering. People were congregated in the yard, none of whom made any attempt to welcome Sarah in and introduce her to others. She waited awkwardly, looking around for the designated greeter. And then a thought came into her head. Maybe I am not welcome here. Sarah started entertaining this thought a bit. Maybe this is a closed group, and people are sad that the former owners are no longer here. Maybe I don't fit in with this group of people. The more she thought about it, the more she believed her initial thought. Next, Sarah experienced an emotion: discomfort. Sarah felt uncomfortable standing there in that backyard with a group of strangers who probably didn't want to get to know her. So, she turned and walked right back out.

What happened here? First, a believed thought (I am not welcome here) then a strong emotion (discomfort) and finally a behavior (leaving the happy hour). This configuration of thought leading to feeling and then to behavior exemplifies how our experiences are processed on the inside.

Now it is entirely possible that the neighbor in charge of welcoming newcomers was momentarily unavailable, in the kitchen pouring a drink or visiting the restroom. If Sarah would have waited a bit longer, she may have been greeted, and the story would have had a happy ending. However, the fatal mistake happened when Sarah chose to believe her initial thought, maybe you are not welcome here.

Recently, I saw a large red bumper sticker that read, "Don't believe everything you think." That one-line sentence highlights a profound truth and hints at a large part of our suffering as human beings. We believe that our thoughts are reality-based facts that transmit certainty. Consequently, we create our own suffering.

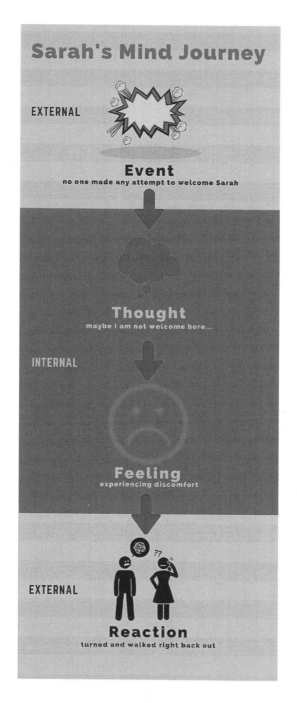

Unhelpful Thinking Styles

Difficult emotions are often preceded by thoughts that can be categorized as unhelpful. In fact, there is a list of common ways of thinking that have been linked to mental health issues such as anxiety and depression. It seems that our minds quite automatically deploy these negative ways of thinking. Which of these unhelpful thinking styles do you use?

1. **Filtering:** You pay attention to negative events or details and magnify those while filtering out the positive. For example, when I received twenty positive end-of-semester evaluations from my students and two negative evaluations, I only "see" the negative feedback and thus I wonder if perhaps I am an ineffective teacher.

2. **Black-and-White Thinking:** No gray area here. Either/or thinking leaves no place for the middle ground. I either do this perfectly right or I am a failure. I either exercise in the gym or not at all. My partner is insensitive; therefore, he must not love me.

3. **Overgeneralization:** We use a single piece of evidence to draw a general conclusion. For example, you tried to meditate once, it didn't feel relaxing, therefore meditation is just not your thing. After the first interview, you didn't get a return call, thus you must be bad at interviewing.

4. **Jumping to Conclusions or Fortune Telling:** We assume that we know what another person is thinking or feeling. Also, we believe we can predict what is going to happen. "If I go to this party, I will feel out-of-place." "He stepped over the trash bag on his way out the door because he is hoping I will take care

of it." "I can see by the look on his face that my friend thinks I am boring."

5. **Catastrophizing:** Blowing things out of proportion is another unhelpful way of thinking. One might notice a mark on the skin and through exaggeration come to believe that it's the first sign of skin cancer. A friend didn't stop by as planned, so she is probably not interested in growing the friendship.

6. **Personalization:** Whatever another person does, says or feels is directly related to me. This thinking style can also manifest itself through taking responsibility for events that really are not your fault. "My colleague is in a bad mood today; he is probably mad that I came to work later than him." "Since I didn't help her with homework, she thinks I don't care about her." "This person cut me off because he is frustrated that I drive slowly."

7. **Emotional Reasoning:** "If I feel it, it must be true." Emotional reasoning is a certain thinking style in which we believe that our feelings are facts. Whatever one currently feels is held to be true because it "feels" like truth. I feel like a failure; therefore, it must be true that I am a failure. I feel anxious, therefore there must be a real threat. However, I do realize that just because I feel anxious getting on a roller coaster doesn't really mean that the roller coaster is a threat to my life.

8. **Chain Thinking:** Link by link, we allow our thinking-train to take us down a dark track. Inevitably, we wind up picturing doomsday or worst-case scenarios. "If I don't get this promotion, it's more likely that I will get fired, and if I get fired I can't pay the bills, and then I end up on the streets."

9. **"Shoulds" and "Musts":** This type of rigid verbiage can rob one of flexibility and delay the process of adapting to the current reality. Charles Darwin spoke about the importance

of adaptability in survival and endurance. "Should" statements often create unrealistic expectations of oneself and others and consequently lead to disappointment. "I should be able to do this right the first time"; "I shouldn't get anxious"; "I am adult, I should be able to be on the plane without fear."

10. **Disqualifying the Positive:** You did something well, but you convince yourself that anyone would have achieved it, or that it really doesn't count. This thinking style has you automatically overlook positive actions or events. "Most people are good at organizing, it's not a big deal, besides, I could be better at it too."

Decluttering the Mind

I love to read and am always interested in new thought-provoking books. I routinely check the current bestseller lineup. A few months ago, a book on the international bestseller list caught my eye: *The Life Changing Magic of Tidying Up: The Japanese Art of Decluttering and Organizing*. The author, Marie Kondo, introduces people to the idea that living a life surrounded by possessions that bring us joy will ultimately lead to lasting happiness and mental health. Of course, this means getting rid of a lot of unnecessary stuff that crams our drawers and covers all surfaces of the home. Marie offers a simply step-by-step approach to letting go, which I modified to fit my model of psychological well-being.

Step 1: Approach an item in your home, for example, a vase.

Step 2: Ask yourself the question, "Does this vase bring me joy?"

- o If the answer is an immediate and resounding YES, the vase gets to stay one of your possessions. If the answer is NO, you move on to step 3.

Step 3: Ask yourself the question, "Does the vase fulfill a purpose?"

- o If the answer is YES, the vase gets to stay. If the answer is NO, you move on to step 4.

Step 4: You communicate gratitude for the item for the time it did bring you joy or serve a purpose and then let it go (think donation pile!).

The goal is to declutter your home and achieve more space. Most of us can sense a relationship between clutter in our physical space and mental angst or anxiety. It feels liberating to let go of disorder.

So how do we declutter the mind? We can follow the same approach. Our minds are often littered with mental noise and a multitude of thoughts. Once you are aware of the mental mess going on in your mind, follow these steps:

Step 1: Notice a thought. "What am I thinking right now?"

Step 2: Ask yourself the question: "Does this thought bring me joy?"

- o If the answer is an immediate and resounding YES, the thought gets to stay in your awareness. If the answer is NO, you move on to step 3.

Step 3: Ask yourself the question, "What purpose does this thought serve?"

- o For example, if the thought is "My boss called but didn't leave a message, and that means I am probably fired," the purpose of that thought (as with most anxiety-induced thoughts) is to prepare you for worst-case scenario.

Step 4: You communicate gratitude to your mind for creating this thought. "Thank you for trying to prepare me for worst-case scenario," and then let go of the thoughts by focusing your attention elsewhere.

The intent behind this approach is to begin changing your relationship with your mind. David Foster Wallace offers the following poignant quote:

"The mind is a wonderful servant but a terrible master."

In essence, this quote challenges all of us to stop allowing the mind to be the boss over our experience. A Buddhist friend of mine shared that, within his Buddhist community, people refer to the mind as a horse. We ride this horse but have no control over it. If the horse wants to stop and eat grass, it stops and eats grass. If it feels like galloping down that meadow, it does just that and we are only along for the ride.

Meditation, psychotherapy, mindfulness practices and reading this book—all these methods provide instructions on becoming the master over your mind.

Therapy Tip

Use coping thoughts to convert the mind to a healthy living space.

Practice: Working with Unhelpful Thoughts: Catch, Classify, Convert

----

The first step of transforming your mind into a healthy living space is to catch unhelpful thoughts as they pop into your mind. Subsequently, classify or label the thought with the help of the unhelpful thinking style list. If you notice that you are engaging in chain thinking, moving from a rather harmless thought to worst-case scenario, stop yourself. Say, "Hold on, what's going on here? Ah, it is my mind doing chain thinking." Next, you convert the negative thought into a coping thought. Have a list of go-to coping thoughts that you can readily recall when the mind is spinning with noise. A client of mine was prepared for the mind's dark thoughts. As soon as the familiar gloomy belief appeared, she used her conversion technique.

- **Negative thought:** "I am a horrible parent because I have thoughts of hitting my child."
- **Coping thought:** "I'm a loving parent who gets worried about thoughts of hitting my child."
- **Negative Thought:** "Germs are everywhere, I will get sick."
- **Coping Thought:** "I am a healthy person who is afraid of getting sick."

I can't handle this. ➡ It isn't easy, but I will get through this.
- My anxiety always goes away eventually.
- I expect my fear to rise, but I can manage it.
- No one is perfect. Progress not perfection.
- Anxiety is a feeling; it doesn't mean anything. This "feeling" has been wrong before.
- Stay focused on this one step. This is all I have to manage.

Practice: Thought Stopping

This technique can be useful for interrupting reoccurring worries and obsessive or intrusive thinking or rumination.

Step 1: Notice that a worry-thought is playing in the mind.

Step 2: Pull up the image of a big, red, shining STOP sign.

Step 3: Shout mentally to yourself, or out loud if possible, "STOP" or "CANCEL."

(Optional—Use with Caution)

Step 4: Place a rubber band around your wrist and snap it each time the unhelpful thought causes you distress. For some people, the pairing of mild discomfort can help shift the mind out of a worrying mindset.

6 I Let Go

A senior monk and a junior monk were traveling together. At one point, they came to a river with a strong current. As the monks were preparing to cross the river, they saw a very young and beautiful woman also attempting to cross. The young woman asked if they could help her cross to the other side.

The two monks glanced at one another because they had taken vows not to touch a woman. Then, without a word, the older monk picked up the woman, carried her across the river, placed her gently on the other side, and carried on his journey.

The younger monk couldn't believe what had just happened. After rejoining his companion, he was speechless, and an hour passed without a word between them. Two more hours passed, then three; finally, the younger monk could contain himself any longer, and blurted out, "As monks, we are not permitted to touch a woman; how could you then carry that woman on your shoulders?"

The older monk looked at him and replied, "Brother, I set her down on the other side of the river; why are you still carrying her?"

What to Let Go of

Often human suffering is connected to our unwillingness to let go. A short time ago, I read a story that took place in an Asian country. The story described how certain ethnic groups capture local monkeys. In some larger cities, monkeys can become a pest, often stealing food in urban markets. Capture and relocation is one way of dealing with the overpopulation. Communities have discovered an effective and humane technique which involves hollowing out several coconuts, dropping a sweet treat into the fruit, drilling a small hole into the top and waiting for the scent to draw in the primates. Once a monkey reaches into the coconut and makes a fist around the treat, the hole is no longer large enough for monkey to get his balled fist out. The animal is not able to let go of the treat and run away into the safety of the jungle. The monkeys sit there trapped by their unwillingness to let go.

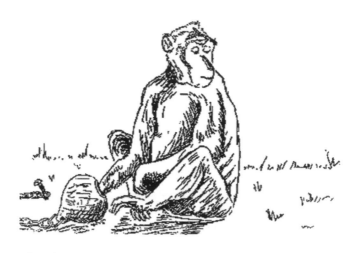

What has you trapped? What are you unwilling to let go of? What does the treat represent in your life? Expectations, desires, past hurts, thoughts, fears, people or possessions? Whatever it is for you, it's probably keeping you from experiencing inner peace on some level. You may or may not be aware of this dynamic occurring in your body and mind.

Let's look at a couple of "treats" that can cause a lot of emotional suffering when held onto for too long.

Perfection

Striving for perfection can often set us up for failure. The standards we set for ourselves are usually so much higher than standards we have for others. Perfectionism quickly leads to self-doubt and elevates fear of disapproval. Striving for progress, on the other hand, encourages and rewards growth. A growth-mindset helps us bounce back from mistakes as we perceive shortcomings not as unacceptable errors but as opportunities for our own personal evolution. Repeat this mantra often: Progress not perfection.

Rumination/Worry

The UK healthcare provider Benenden Health conducted a survey on worrying which revealed that the average person spends about five years of his or her life worrying about issues such as finances, health, family members, getting old and his or her love life. What would your life look like without the habit of worrying? For one, you'd have more mental energy to spend elsewhere.

Comparison

A fast-track way to feeling lousy is when we compare ourselves to others. Often social media is just that: an epic compare-ism machine. We evaluate our own present ordinary experience alongside the larger-than-life photo of our friend's epic girls' night out. Consequently, feelings of inferiority and inadequacy arise. Before that picture popped up on our device, we were actually feeling just fine. Thich Nhat Hanh, a modern-day Zen master, reminds us that "To be beautiful means to be yourself. You don't need to be accepted by others. You need to accept yourself." In an effort to be more mindful of letting go of comparison, perhaps instead of checking social media, use that time to make a list of things you like about yourself.

Guilt

The feeling of guilt comes up when we think we have gone against an internal value. If you feel guilty a lot, it probably means you care about being the best version of yourself. However, some of us habitually feel guilty; it's a habit of self-doubt. Therefore, it's important to differentiate habit-guilt from helpful-guilt. Helpful-guilt directs these feelings towards healthy self-improvement. Use Socratic questions to reflect on your experience of guilt.

1. Did I really do something wrong here?
2. What's the evidence for or against it?
3. Am I basing this guilt-based thought on facts or feelings?
4. Could my guilt-based thought be an exaggeration of what's true?
5. Might other people have a different interpretation of this situation?

Insecurities

The most harmful repercussions of feeling insecure can be felt in our relationships. The thought, "something is wrong with me" or "I am not good enough" can paralyze our social skills. We assume others have already cast their judgments upon us, so we disengage or become offensive. No one has the skill to mind-read. You have the power to override thoughts of insecurity. "Nothing is wrong with me, I am simply feeling insecure"; "This insecurity is a feeling that will pass" or "I am getting more confident every day." The next time you are in a situation that brings up feelings of self-doubt, take a deep breath, visualize what a confident you would look like, and move forward replicating that image. You may even want to pretend playing a role of a confident, strong person, just like actors have to do for their jobs. Fake it till you make it—it really works!

Anger

In session with some of my younger clients, we often draw an internal volcano. The internal volcano is a metaphor for our anger. When a volcano erupts, it can be a scary show: all that smoke and lava combined with an intense heat. Once the eruption has quieted some, it's essential to look a bit deeper under the surface. Anger is an exterior or secondary emotion. Underneath our anger, other more primary emotions provide the fuel, usually a hurt or a fear. What am I afraid of—where is the hurt here?

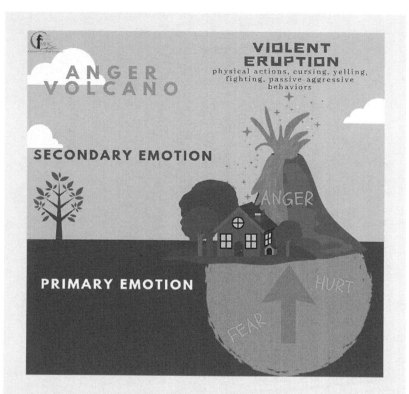

Bob came to counseling for anger management. He would get so angry at his wife that he would hurtle a slew of cruel words in her direction. Bob didn't really have an anger problem. He was deeply hurt that his wife wasn't valuing his contributions at home. This insight helped both partners voice their needs to each other, consequently helping some of Bob's anger to subside.

Letting Go Like Nature

It's all about letting go, isn't it? In some way, we are born to let go. Our final destination is the ultimate letting go, namely, death. Accordingly, each evening as we fall asleep, we are letting go of a day, which is never to return. Quite similar is the journey of having and raising children. Parenting is a unique job: We are working ourselves out of a job from day one. Each day, as children slowly but surely become more independent, parents begin letting go. Our child's first step, first day of school, first time driving, and first graduation are all stages with the goal of releasing them to the world.

Each time the fall season comes around, I feel a bit melancholy, not ready to say goodbye to the warmth and golden glow of late summer. Yet the trees seem undisturbed: it seems easy for them to let go. There is no struggle. The trees know when to release what they no longer need. In their wisdom, trees know they are not dying; they are just letting go of what isn't theirs to hold on to. What does each falling leaf represent in your life? An expectation, a need for approval, a personal failure, a "should-have-been"?

The less trees carry into the winter, the better. Holding on would kill them. The releasing is life-giving. I ask myself, as

83

I watch each leaf drift through the air, what do I need to let fall away this season to make room for new growth?

The Case of Danny

Danny, a middle-aged woman, had a full life. Her husband's career success had allowed her to stay home as she was raising her four children. Just a few years after the youngest took off to college, Danny became a grandmother and happily stepped into her new role. Her days became over-filled with childcare duties, Bible study, volunteering, and a multitude of household chores. Danny sought help for feeling overwhelmed, irritable, sad and constantly jumpy.

In the second session, I explained to Danny that she was suffering from generalized anxiety disorder. Consequently, we discussed necessary lifestyle changes to improve her ability to manage the anxiety. Danny's body language spoke of ambiguity. I shifted my approach.

"Danny, let's say I am your primary-care physician giving you the news that you have Type II diabetes. As you know, people with diabetes can live long and productive lives if one is willing to make a few lifestyle changes such as dietary modifications, increased exercise, and medication management. The same is true for anxiety. Just as diabetes is a disease affecting your blood sugar, anxiety is an illness affecting your emotions and mood. Certain lifestyle changes can make anxiety more manageable."

This comparison helped Danny release some of the stigma she associated with anxiety. Danny started working on a few lifestyle changes related to letting go. Here is her list:

- **Let go of overscheduling:** Stop running from one appointment or activity to the next without having an extended break.

- **Let go of saying "yes.":** Remember that every time you are saying "yes" to something or someone, you are also saying "no" to what you may need (hint: down-time).

- **Let go of "shoulds" and comparisons:** When you "should" yourself, you are not listening to what your body or mind actually needs to create calm.

Danny made peace with the fact that she suffered from anxiety. Comparing her schedule with her friend's—someone who was able to run around all day without feeling anxious—is not helpful because that's not Danny's reality. She also practiced asking herself the following question throughout her day:

What can I let go of right now that's going to create a bit more space?

That inquiry assisted Danny in letting go of appointments, duties, or expectations to support her endeavor to create a mentally healthier lifestyle.

Practice: Letting Go of Rumination

This step-by-step process can be useful for letting go of constant rumination.

Step 1: Take pause to do some deeper investigation. What is the deepest fear surrounding the rumination? Get your thoughts on paper; journaling is a useful way to identify the underlying fears.

Step 2: Play the "Worst Case Scenario" game. Once we play it out in our imagination, we may realize that we can actually handle the worst-case scenario if it were to happen. Human beings are astoundingly resilient. So are you!

Step 3: Think about what you can control in this situation. Make a 3-step action plan for what you can do to help that situation. Let go of what you can't control. For example, if you ruminate on losing your job, your 3-step action plan might include:
1) updating your resume
2) speaking with your boss on how to improve your work performance
3) taking continuing education classes to make yourself more marketable

What happens next is not in your control—let it go.

(Tip: A change of scenery can do wonders for interrupting the ruminating mind.)

Practice: Letting-Go Rituals

Letting go often does not work if it stays a mere intellectual exercise. For letting go to sink in, we sometimes need to engage in a physical ritual. The following suggestions have been used by numerous clients.

○ Walk a Labyrinth. Labyrinths have been used for centuries as a form of prayer or meditation. One follows a circular path that eventually leads to a center point. Perhaps walk it with the intention of letting go once you arrive in the center. For more information on labyrinths and how to experience them, see https://labyrinthlocator.com.

○ Burn it. Perhaps find a suitable object that represents what you need to let go of. In silence and solitude, give the object to the fire. This can also be done by composing a letting-go letter that consequently gets burned. Fire is a powerful symbol of purification and renewal.

o Go on a favorite hiking trail. Fill your backpack with a few large, heavy rocks. Be clear what those rocks represent for you. Hike with the heavy pack for a good long time. When the time is right, and an appropriate location has been found, toss each rock far away from your body. Be clear what you are letting go of with each throw. A splash in the water might enhance the experience. As you hike back, notice the lightness of your backpack.

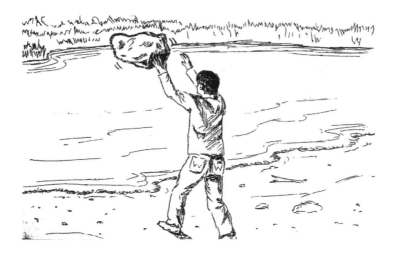

7 I Mindfully Accept

Once there was a Chinese farmer who worked his poor farm together with his son and their horse. When the horse ran off one day, neighbors came to say, "How unfortunate for you!" The farmer replied, "Maybe yes, maybe no."

When the horse returned, followed by a herd of wild horses, the neighbors gathered around and exclaimed, "What good luck for you!" The farmer stayed calm and replied, "Maybe yes, maybe no."

While trying to tame one of wild horses, the farmer's son fell and broke his leg. He had to rest up and couldn't help with the farm chores. "How sad for you," the neighbors cried. "Maybe yes, maybe no," said the farmer.

Shortly thereafter, a neighboring army threatened the farmer's village. All the young men in the village were drafted to fight the invaders. Many died. But the farmer's son had been left out of the fighting because of his broken leg. People said to the farmer, "What a good thing your son couldn't fight!" "Maybe yes, maybe no," was all the farmer said.

The Judgmental Nature of the Mind

The story of the Chinese farmer illustrates numerous philosophical truths. Fundamentally, this tale brings to our awareness the never-ending judgmental nature of the mind. Often without our knowledge, our mind has already spun numerous judgments about the person, place or thing that has entered consciousness. That person looks rich; he's probably a lawyer dressed like that. That child is so obnoxious; she probably doesn't get disciplined enough at home. I don't like meditation; it's so boring. You get the point. The mind constantly places thoughts into categories of good and bad. For illustration sake, try saying the following sentence to yourself:

"I am perfect."

What happened when you said those three words to yourself? Inevitably, your mind creates some judgment around those words such as "Well, that just makes me laugh, I am nowhere near perfect. There was that time when I...." You were merely asked to say three words back to yourself, but what most of us did is immediately judge those words. Thus, is the nature of the mind. There isn't a whole lot we can do about it other than become aware of this tendency and perhaps remind ourselves that judgments aren't reality—they are simply creations of the mind. The farmer from the story wasn't as quick to jump to conclusions based on his critical mind. He was able to take a step back and remember that life is a blend of complex, interwoven circumstances that demands adaptation and flexibility.

Mindful Acceptance

A Buddhist teacher once explained to me that the Buddhist version of grace can be understood as one's ability to fully accept each moment with compassion and non-judgment. Of course, this is easy with the good moments. When a loved-one holds you close and professes his or her love, that moment is readily welcomed in. However, this also means welcoming the difficult moments: for example, the instant you receive a cancer diagnosis, or your teenager is caught taking drugs. Acceptance of these types of crisis moments take a lifetime of practice. It is important to differentiate acceptance from approval here. Acceptance of a crisis-moment does not mean approving or being resigned to it. It is more about acknowledging and allowing pain and suffering to be here right now. It's not about liking unpleasant emotions but acknowledging them and no longer fighting our internal experience. For this intent and purpose, let's uncover ways of making micro-progress towards mindful acceptance.

Baby-steps towards mindful acceptance:

o Allowing difficult feelings to be here. This doesn't mean you won't take action to help yourself manage these emotions later.

o Anger or sadness has a right to be part of your experience just as much as joy and excitement.

o Saying "yes" to your anxiety or anger supports the natural waning process of feelings.

o "I am noticing the feeling of anxiety right now, nothing is wrong with feeling anxious, and it will eventually dissipate".

o "This moment is okay just the way it is."

Some of my worst parenting moments involved my two children fighting. This usually included two rather loud voices in the back of the car arguing over who got to rest their arm in the middle section. Yeah, really! Consequently, I got sucked into the discord by being assigned the job of referee. Amidst rising frustration and impatience, I would, at times, explode.

Mindful acceptance of this situation would look like this:

o   I accept what I feel right now; I won't deny my feelings.

o   It is rough to be a parent sometimes. Frustration is a normal part of parenting.

o   Acceptance first, change later. Once we are all in a more positive state of mind, we can discuss ways of dealing with the situation in a healthier way.

o   Can I say "yes" to this moment of discomfort?

o   Can I allow myself to experience whatever is happening right now rather than wishing for a different reality?

The Antidote: Curiosity

One way to help your mind move away from being judgmental is through the use of curiosity. The beloved kids book character, Curious George, is an endearing little monkey whose spirit of inquiry motivates him to see the world as an adventure. What if you could adopt George's playful curiosity when exploring your internal experience?

Becoming curious

- What is going on with me right now?
- How do I feel emotionally?
- What kind of thoughts are going through my head?
- What does my body feel like in this moment?
- Can I watch my internal struggle without judging it?
- Can I experience the pain without drowning in it?
- Can I allow the hurt without becoming it?

Drop the Storyline

The moment my children started arguing on the car drive home, my whole body started to tense up. I notice how I was clenching my jaw and furrowing my forehead. My body was saying "Mayday, Mayday, approaching threatening situation." Hoping to release some of the tension in my upper body, I began taking deep, full breaths. Consequently, I became curious about the stories that my mind was creating around the drama unfolding in my car. The storyline went something like this: "These kids are really badly behaved. You did not do a good job raising them. And you call yourself a therapist? You can't even control your own children." Reflecting on the toxicity of those thoughts, I was able to drop the storyline and replace it with more helpful contemplations such as "It's normal that siblings fight; every parent has been in this situation. Give yourself a break— parenting can be hard."

Here is 6-step formula to put it all together and help manage difficult emotions:

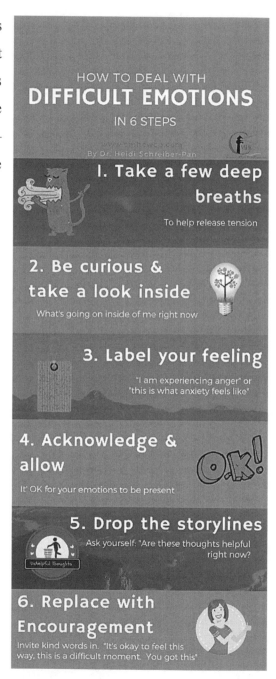

HOW TO DEAL WITH
DIFFICULT EMOTIONS
IN 6 STEPS
By Dr. Heidi Schreiber-Pan

1. Take a few deep breaths
To help release tension

2. Be curious & take a look inside
What's going on inside of me right now

3. Label your feeling
"I am experiencing anger" or "this is what anxiety feels like"

4. Acknowledge & allow
It' OK for your emotions to be present

5. Drop the storylines
Ask yourself: "Are these thoughts helpful right now?
Unhelpful Thoughts

6. Replace with Encouragement
Invite kind words in. "It's okay to feel this way, this is a difficult moment. You got this"

Practice: Dialog with Rumi

Jalal al-Din Rumi was a 13th century poet and mystic whose literary work continues to influence contemporary philosophers and spiritual leaders. One of Rumi's best loved poems is titled "The Guest House." Read this poem twice. Next, take some time to ponder the reflection questions.

This being human is a guest house.
Every morning a new arrival.
A joy, a depression, a meanness,
some momentary awareness comes
as an unexpected visitor.

Welcome and entertain them all!
Even if they are a crowd of sorrows,
who violently sweep your house
empty of its furniture,
still, treat each guest honorably.

He may be clearing you out
for some new delight.

The dark thought, the shame, the malice.
meet them at the door laughing and invite them in.

Be grateful for whatever comes.
because each has been sent
as a guide from beyond.
-Rumi

1. What unexpected visitors have shown up at your guest house lately?

2. How do you habitually respond to "visitors" whom you don't like?

3. Is it possible to welcome in emotions? If yes, how?

4. What make up your "crowd of sorrows"? Compose a list.

5. In what way can you perceive difficult emotions as honorable guest?

6. Rumi speaks about "clearing you out for some new delight." What do you make of this statement? Can challenging emotions be beneficial, even valuable?

7. Rumi suggests that the dark thought, the shame, the malice could be sent as a guide from beyond. Is this perspective consistent with your religious/spiritual set of beliefs?

I Mindfully Accept

8

Self-*Care,* Not Self-*ish*

A few years ago, I attended a Tara Brach workshop where she shared a story of a renowned Hawaiian healer. This healer was celebrated throughout the islands as a man of great wisdom and healing power. When he reached the end of life, one of his longtime students ask him to share the secret of his success. "How did you help so many people? How did you help them find happiness?" The healer replied, "All I did was guide people to turn toward themselves and say I love you, I forgive you and I am sorry. When people can genuinely do that for themselves, true healing begins."

Self-Care Not Self-ish

A lot of people struggle with caring for themselves. It often comes more naturally to look after our children or ailing parents. That's what we are supposed to do, right? Well, yes and no. Most of us want to live our lives according to a moral framework that has been passed down to us by our parents, faith traditions or cultural standards. Often such moral principles applaud selflessness and personal sacrifice. There is nothing wrong with serving others: in fact, a researcher named Borgonovi suggests that people who volunteer report better health and more happiness than people who do not volunteer.

However, being other-focused can also create anxiety, stress and resentment. How do we make sure that assisting others does not generate these types of negative emotions? First of all, it is absolutely essential to care for ourselves. If our needs have not been met, we are entering into relationships with a tank half empty.

Here is an example of self-care activities that some people find rejuvenating.

- o *Getting a massage*
- o *Gardening*
- o Running or jogging
- o Walking
- o Communing with nature
- o Working out
- o Yoga

Taking time out of the busyness of your day to engage in these types of self-care practices has positive repercussions. Not only do we feel more replenished, we are often more emotionally balanced. Therefore, self-care is a prerequisite for caring and helping others.

Certain individuals will insist that getting a massage instead of volunteering at church is inheritably selfish. I argue, however, that your family, your church and your workplace desire the best version of yourself. Intentional self-care is an effort to send love, care and respect to the person we spend most of our time with: ourselves. Remember a time when you felt irritable and snapped at a family member? Chances are that you were lacking in self-care that day. How would our lives change if we would stop on occasion and ask ourselves the following question?

What is it that I need right now?

Prior to takeoff, air travel personnel will instruct all passengers in the event of air pressure imbalance to place an oxygen mask on oneself first before helping a child. Of course, it makes sense that if this father doesn't care for his oxygen, he may faint before being able to assist his son. This reference speaks truth to the significance of self-care in our daily lives.

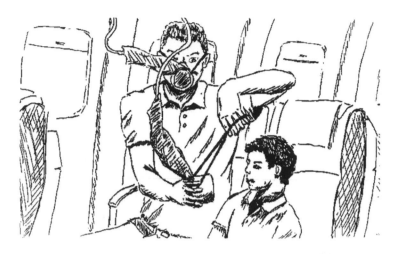

Experiment with substituting the world selfish with the word self-care in your vocabulary, particularly in your internal dialogue. *"Am I being selfish when saying 'no' to this request?"* *"Am I caring for myself by saying 'no' to this request?"*

> *"Self-care is never a selfish act—it is simply good stewardship of the only gift I have, the gift I was put on earth to offer to others."* -Parker Palmer

Therapy Tip

Did you grow up in a home where your emotional needs were not met? If yes, then it's likely that you learned to place your own needs on the back burner. You now have an extraordinary opportunity to make things right. Care for that (inner) child of yours. Do you believe in child advocacy? If yes, then start with the kid inside.

Self-Compassion

Kristin Neff, researcher and author, has pioneered the concept of self-compassion. In her well-known Ted Talk, she distinguishes self-esteem from self-compassion. She repeatedly highlights the positive effect of bringing kindness to one's experience as we practice self-compassion. Self-esteem follows a different agenda. It is based on evaluations and self-worth, the goal being to eradicate insecurities. Dr. Neff believes what our culture really needs is an emphasis on self-compassion.

Think back to your elementary or middle school days. Did you have a teacher who was harsh and authoritarian, a teacher who was impatient and quick to point out failures? In middle school, I had a math teacher like that. She frequently let the class know how disappointed she was in the overall class effort. Moreover, she picked me to solve complex math problems on the board in front of the class. I was struggling with math at the time and remember cringing whenever I would walk to that class. Self-doubt and mistrust in my ability to do calculations increased. At the end of that school year, I was convinced that I was bad at math. A year later, I had the most wonderful English teacher. Mr. Beck believed in me, envisioning my potential. He would say, "I can't wait to see what amazing things you'll write about in your next essay." After receiving a low score on a test, he would encourage me with words of affirmation. I wanted to do well in his class to prove him correct that I really was a success. As I moved on to high school, he told me to make sure to inform him once I achieved my PhD degree.

Which teacher created a better learning environment? Of course, it was Mr. Beck. He was my personal cheerleader, quick to praise and encourage. What teacher are you to yourself? A lot of us engage in consistent self-critique. "Ah there you go again—you just don't learn." "What's wrong with you? You've been in therapy for a year and you still get anxious." "Why can't you be more like Jeff who has tons of friends and is always in a positive mood?"

Self-compassion turns the volume down on the inner critic while at the same time amplifying the internal cheerleader.

The How of Self-Compassion

In the summer of 2017, I had the difficult task of dropping my oldest son off at college. He settled on a school that was exactly 1,694 miles from home, so not exactly a place that you can visit on a whim. As I was getting ready to drop him off, my emotions began to storm. I quickly said my goodbyes and jumped in the car. Within ten minutes of leaving the campus, I found myself sobbing. It was truly upsetting to leave this child behind, whom I had nurtured for 18 years. Thus, I decided this was a good time to give myself a dose of self-compassion.

Kristin Neff provides us with a formula to accomplish this tough assignment.

1. **Check in with the stories of the mind:** When I shifted my attention to the stories that my mind was creating, I heard this: "What's wrong with you? You should be happy for him. This is a normal part of growing up—get over it! Why is this so hard for you? You are probably overly attached." Needless to say, these thoughts created lots of suffering within me. After a moment of reflection, I chuckled at the falsehoods my mind was spawning and said out loud, "These stories are unhelpful and untrue. Be gone!"

2. **Allow the pain to be there:** We often rush to placate our sorrow. Subsequently, the pain is not able to come to its full expression. Leftover, stored pain can have a long-term aftereffect. "Heidi, this hurts and that is OK. It is normal to feel pain at this loss. I am going to allow the pain to be as big as it needs to be." Therefore, I permitted the tears, the sobbing, the pain to be there all the way to the airport, which was a two-hour drive.

3. **Remember others' suffering:** Often when we are hurting, we believe that nobody can understand the depth of our pain. We feel isolated in our suffering from the outside world. Therefore, I reminded myself of the truth that in this very moment many other mothers were grieving the loss of their college-bound child—just like me. That awareness allowed me to step out of isolation and into connection with others.

4. **Create a physical representation of compassion:** It is essential that we conclude these action-steps with a physical representation of self-compassion: a bodily touch directed at yourself as a sign of sending kindness toward your own pain. Perhaps this consists of placing your hands over your heart or a gentle embrace as your hands stroke

the opposite shoulders. Maybe this gesture could be a tender framing of the face with both hands. Driving in the car, I simply reached over and softly patted my left hand and whispered, "There, there."

End-of-Life Lesson

As a doctorate student of counseling psychology, my second-year internship took place in a hospice setting. Part of my role as a counselor there was to be with families as their loved-ones were dying. Rather quickly, I came to understand that it did not matter what racial or socio-economic background the dying person was from. The only things that really matter for any person at the end are

- relationship with others,
- relationship with self,
- relationship with higher being/spirituality.

It was my experience that, as people were preparing to transition out of their lives, what brought meaning to the dying consisted of these three significant relationships (others, self and spirit). The last time I checked, the mortality rate around here constitutes 100%. Therefore, if we are all heading in that direction, what are we doing daily to nurture these three relationships? At the very end, we even must let go of the relationships with others, so we can move forward and complete our final letting go. That leaves us with two: relationship with self and relationship with spirit. If these are the last and most significant connections that will see us safely across the great divide, we must make them a priority. Self-compassion is a beautiful way to start building a loving bond with yourself.

Practice: Self-Care Practice Inventory

Consider this list and circle the practices that you would like to begin or continue doing as part of your self-care plan. Commit to integrating at least one item into your daily routine.

- Gardening
- Running, jogging, or walking
- Communing with Nature
- Working out
- Yoga
- Meeting up with friends
- Going out to lunch or dinner
- Taking a nap
- Engaging in a hobby
- Meditating or praying
- Attending a retreat
- Seeing a therapist
- Doing a technology fast
- Decluttering the home
- Writing down thoughts, a.k.a. journaling
- Going to bed earlier
- Joining a book club
- Getting massages regularly
- Saying "no" to certain commitments
- Findings ways to laugh
- Taking breaks through the workday
- Enjoying quiet
- Volunteering
- Singing or dancing
- Keeping the Sabbath (e.g., dedicate one day to rest)

Practice: Self-Care Plan

Use the information from this chapter to create a detailed self-care plan. If it doesn't get scheduled, it usually doesn't happen. Get these practices on your calendar.

A wheel only works if it is well-balanced. That means all six areas of your self-care wheel need to receive an equal amount of your attention. Look at all the categories: Are there a few that you do a better job of nourishing than others?

SELF-CARE
WHEEL

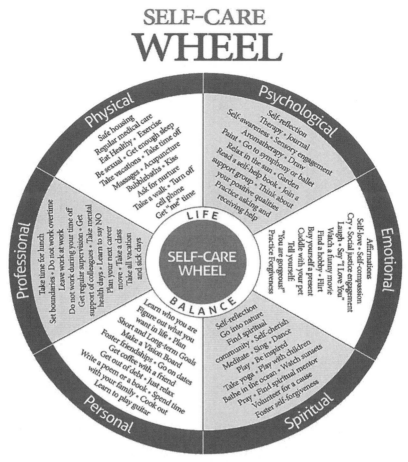

This Self-Care Wheel was inspired by and adapted from "Self-Care Assessment Worksheet" from *Transforming the Pain: A Workbook on Vicarious Traumatization* by Saakvitne, Pearlman & Staff of TSI/CAAP (Norton, 1996). Created by Olga Phoenix Project: Healing for Social Change (2013). Dedicated to all trauma professionals worldwide.

www.OlgaPhoenix.com

Practice: Self-Compassion Exercise adapted from Kristin Neff

---

1. Bring to mind an image of yourself as a young child. What age comes to mind? Can you picture yourself? What are you wearing?

2. Imagine that the little girl or boy from your imagination has experienced a failure of some kind or is struggling with something

3. What would you say to her or him? Most likely it would be words of encouragement and reassurance: "Hey, it's okay, that happens sometimes. You got this!" This is often the direct opposite of the way we speak to ourselves, right? As we practice self-compassion, it is very helpful to think of our young, tender child that still lives inside our memories.

4. Find a picture of yourself as a child. Place it on your bathroom mirror, the dashboard of your car, any place that receives your attention frequently throughout the day. The photograph serves as a reminder to treat yourself with the utmost kindheartedness, just like you would that cute little kid from the picture.

113

9 Setting Boundaries

Perhaps you are familiar with the well-known story from the New Testament about the Good Samaritan. Jesus shares this parable in response to the question "Who is your neighbor?" Jesus tells of a man who gets robbed, beaten and left for dead at the side of the road. Several people, including clergy, pass by the man without offering to help. At this point in the story, Jesus introduces us to the Good Samaritan, a person whose Samaritan heritage was seen as hostile from a Jewish perspective. Nevertheless, he felt sorry for the injured man.

"He went to him and bandaged his wounds, pouring oil and wine on him. Then he put the man on his own donkey, brought him to an inn and took care of him. The next day he took out two denari and gave them to the innkeeper. 'Look after him,' he said, 'and when I return, I will reimburse you for any extra expense you may have" (Luke 10:25-16:17 NIV).

Let's imagine there was a Part II to this familiar tale. As the Good Samaritan (a.k.a. Sam) is about to leave, the injured person wakes up, slowly takes in the situation and begs to have a word with Sam. "You aren't leaving me, are you?" asks the injured man. "Well, I have to go and look after my family now, but I have bandaged your wounds, the inn is paid for and you can even stay a few more days to heal. I will reimburse the inn for any extra expenses," he replies. "And I thank you for all of that. However, I still need you right now—I am not well yet, as you can see. Please stay longer." Sam starts to think about it. He really needs to depart right now: His family is already waiting for him, not to mention his business has suffered from his absence. Noticing the Good Samaritan's hesitancy, the injured man continues. "I am still hurting and in pain here and you are thinking about leaving—it's just so selfish of you." Well, I don't want to be selfish, thinks Sam. Thus, he decides to stay. Not long after his decision to stay, Sam experiences a new emotion: resentment. Resentment has replaced his earlier emotions of compassion, kindness and empathy. He becomes increasingly irritable. He wonders what happened: He doesn't like all these negative feelings. The injured person, on the other hand, thoroughly enjoys having found someone to take care of all his needs.

(Story adapted from Henry Cloud and John Sims Townsend, Boundaries: When to Say Yes, When to Say No to Take Control of Your Life. 1992.)

Boundaries

Let's say you and I are standing across from one another. There is about ten feet between us. I instruct you to say "stop" once I have crossed the line into your personal space. I begin walking towards you. I get closer and closer. At some point you say, "Stop." You have just set your physical boundary. As unique individuals, we all say "Stop" at slightly different distances. In some sense, boundaries keep us safe—they provide a form of protection.

Think of your bedroom. You have a clear understanding where your bedroom begins and where your bedroom ends. If someone enters your room and dumps a bunch of dirty laundry on your rug and you start cleaning it up, a boundary violation has occurred. That laundry is not your responsibility, yet you take care of it. People quickly notice that you are "that guy/gal" who takes care of stuff. More laundry ends up in your room.

Now, most of us don't actually allow others' laundry to be deposited in our bedrooms. However, this analogy shines light on other areas in our lives where we take on things that are not our duty.

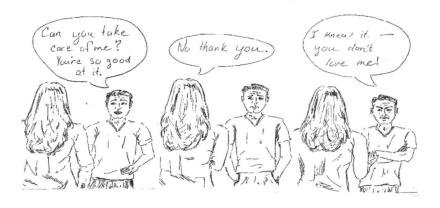

Boundary-Weak Tasha

Tasha was an integral part of the therapy group that met at a local church on Sunday evenings. The other attendees enjoyed Tasha's presence and insight. The group was great at showering each member with encouragement. However, the group was also an excellent accountability partner. Tasha was generally more of a listener, but this week she spoke about a recent struggle that occurred almost every evening at her house. Tasha would spend her afternoons preparing dinner for her family. She loved cooking and took great pride in her ability to create a meal that all four of them enjoyed. Nevertheless, when Tasha called everyone to the table, people wouldn't come. After the third announcement at least ten minutes later, her family members would slowly arrive. By then the food would be cold. This made Tasha furious, yet she never voiced her displeasure from fear of causing conflict. Tasha told the group that she felt disrespected and devalued.

Consequently, the group decided that Tasha had to set limits and enforce boundaries with her family. Her assignment was to let everyone know that she expected people to be on-time for dinner and failing to do so was disrespectful to her efforts to create a family dinner experience. Next, the group told Tasha that after five minutes of nobody showing for dinner, she had to gather up all the food and throw it out. Tasha was appalled by the prospect of wasting food, so she agreed to bring it to the neighbors. She did it! Her family was stunned. They complained and whined about it for over an hour. But the next day, they arrived at the dinner table five minutes early!

Tasha had begun setting boundaries. She communicated how she wanted to be treated, what she could tolerate and what behavior was unacceptable. Tasha found her voice. She was bound to assert her needs.

Tasha grew up the youngest in a family of seven and was the only girl. Her parents were often preoccupied with their oldest child Rick's enormous mood swings. Tasha observed as every family member took on the task of keeping Rick happy and calm. As an adult, she perpetuated the dysfunctional dynamic with her brother that was modeled by her parents. When Rick was unhappy, she would spend hours on the phone being supportive and brainstorming ways to lift him up. Rick would rarely ask about Tasha's life. It was a one-sided relationship that focused exclusively on the well-being of Rick.

After months of therapy, Tasha freed herself from the responsibility of being her brother's caretaker. Rick resented this new version of Tasha, showering his sister with shame and hurtful words. Eventually, Rick realized that his sister was no longer coming to the rescue, so he found Elaine. To this day, Rick and Elaine are in a toxic and unhappy marriage. "I feel sorry for my brother. I am also really sad that I can't have him in my life, but I had to learn to protect myself from his harmful behavior."

Taking Responsibility for Me

In therapy, Tasha discovered that is was not her responsibility to make her brother happy or to fix his situation. Boundaries clarify what our responsibilities are.

You Are Responsible For

o Choices you make

o Your feelings

o Your well-being and happiness

o Creating purpose and meaning in your life

o Your coping strategies

o Your attitude

o Your mindset

You Are NOT Responsible For

o A person's thoughts

o A person's feelings

o A person's happiness

o A person's values

o Other people liking you

o A person's behavior

o A person's choice

o How other's respond to you

Therapy Tip

We can support others' well-being, yet we are not responsible for their happiness.

Boundaries are a tough concept for children to understand yet helping them do so is an essential ingredient of parenting. Part of childrearing is helping developing minds recognize that the choices they make bear natural consequences. When my son was seven years old, he would create elaborate Lego designs. He'd work for hours. One day, he had constructed something similar to the Eiffel Tower with spare Lego pieces littering the floor of our living room. I gently reminded him that dinner time was fast approaching, and the floor needed to be Lego-free within the next ten minutes. I assured him that the Eiffel Tower itself could remain. "I am going to set this timer to help remind you of your chore. You have ten minutes to put all the pieces in the box. However, if you choose not to do that, I will have to clean up your whole set-up, ok?" As the time was ticking away, I spoke a silent prayer: Please make him clean up. I don't want to destroy his creation. "Whoops, now there are only five minutes left on the timer." When the timer rung, I reminded him of the choice he just made and the natural consequence of his action. I think we both cried that afternoon.

What motivated me to follow through that day was a disturbing forethought of my grown son fighting with his wife because he never helps clean up the house.

Healthy Boundaries, Healthy Life

Many people with anxiety have difficulty setting limits, trouble with saying "No." Anxious individuals often submit to the needs of other people. Their lack of attunement and follow-through toward their own needs can create the conditions for the perfect storm. Individuals struggling with stress and anxiety benefit from a less is more lifestyle. Running from one commitment to another without breathing space activates our sympathetic nervous system, leading to a sense of fight-or-flight. Is it possible to protect one's breathing space when saying "no" to others seems unfeasible?

Healthy Boundary Tips:

1. Let others do what they can do for themselves. To empower someone means to provide them with the tools so they can achieve their goals. To enable someone means to support them in perpetuating unhelpful behavior.

2. Respect yourself and demand respect from others. You need to be your own advocate. Voice your needs.

3. Nurture evenhanded relationships. If you are the one who always listens but rarely shares, is the friendship properly balanced?

4. Setting boundaries is part of self-care.

> ## Therapy Tip
>
> *The fear of being selfish can lead to weak boundaries. If you are wondering if you are selfish, rest assured that truly selfish people lack the capacity to entertain that very thought.*

The Bridge – A Boundary Parable

This parable speaks of a man who is contemplating the direction his life is taking. He is unsure about his future. After much contemplation, he achieves great clarity and is excited about the vision he can see for his life. He starts off on the journey to his future.

He must travel to another town where an amazing opportunity has presented itself, but he must get there by the next morning or the opportunity will pass.

He travels many hours, getting more excited about the life he is creating with each step he takes. As the full moon rises, he is alone in his thoughts as he starts crossing a bridge.

The man sees out of the corner of his eye a stranger coming towards him. He thinks the man approaching is putting his hand out to greet him. However, the stranger has the end of a rope in his hand with the other end wound around his waist.

The stranger asks the man to hold the end of the rope. Although perplexed, the man complies.

The stranger asks the man to hold on tight with two hands and then promptly jumps off the bridge toward the swift running deep river below. "Hold on!" the stranger cries.

The free-falling body hurtled the distance of the rope's length, and from the bridge the man abruptly felt the pull. He held tight despite being almost pulled over the side of the bridge.

Peering down at the stranger who was close to oblivion, the man yelled, "What are you trying to do?"

"Just hold tight," said the other.

The man tried to haul the stranger in, but he could not. He could not get enough leverage. His strength was almost perfectly counterbalanced by the other man's weight.

"Why did you do this?" the man called out. "Remember," said the other, "if you let go, I will be lost."

"But I cannot pull you up," the man cried. "Just hold on. I need you," the stranger yells.

The man looked around for help, but no one was near. The man holds on for a while, and then calls, "Please, I cannot hold you. Please climb up."

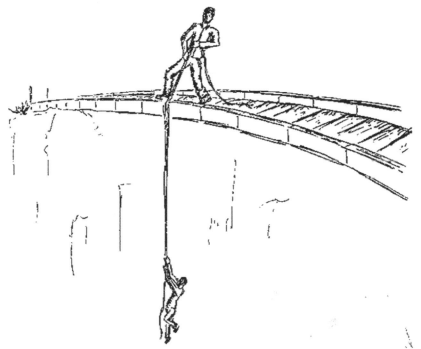

"I am your responsibility," said the other. "Well, I did not ask for it," the man said. The stranger cried, "If you let go, I am lost."

The man tried to invent solutions, like tying the rope to the bridge, but could not find any that would work.

Fearing that his arms could not hold out much longer, he tied the rope around his waist.

He thought if he just waited long enough, someone was bound to come and help pull the stranger up. He waited many hours, but no one came.

"Why did you do this?" he asked again. "Don't you see what you have done? What possible purpose could you have had in mind?"

"Just remember," said the other, "my life is in your hands."

Time passed, and a decision needed to be made. The man could not hold on much longer.

A thought occurred to him. If the stranger hauled himself up and he kept the end steady and pulled a bit, together they could get the stranger back to safety.

But the other wasn't interested.

"You mean you won't help? But I told you I cannot pull you up myself, and I don't think I can hang on much longer either." "You must try," the other shouted back in tears. "If you fail, I die."

More time passed and finally, the point of decision arrived. The man said to the other, "Listen to me. I will not accept the position of choice for your life, only for my own;

the position of choice for your own life I hereby give back to you."

"What do you mean?" the other asked, afraid.

"I mean, simply, it's up to you. You decide which way this ends. I will help you if you help yourself."

"You cannot mean what you say," the other shrieked. "You would not be so selfish. I am your responsibility. What could be so important that you would let someone die? Do not do this to me."

The man stated again, "I will not stand here and hold this rope. If you want to live, you must start moving now, and I will help you. Please, start now."

He waited a few minutes, but there was no change in the tension of the rope. "I accept your choice," the man said, at last, and freed his hands.

(By the late Rabbi Edwin Friedman)

The story is a powerful reminder that we often take on another person's problems. We allow that person to rope us into their world of pain and suffering. Of course, most of us adhere to moral guidelines that motivate us to aid a person in need. It is a virtuous thing to do, within limits. If you feel overwhelmed and consumed by the relationship, it's no longer a virtue but a vice. Also, pay attention to the feeling of resentment. Resentment is a tell-tale sign that a line has been crossed, you have given more than you should have, and boundaries have been violated.

"The first thing you need to learn is that the person who is angry at you for setting boundaries is the one with the problem."

-Drs. Cloud and Townsend

Practice: What's in Your Backpack?

Imagine that you are going for a hike to the top of a mountain. You are so excited to reach the peak. Suddenly, God* appears and says, "Would you be willing to take these things to the top of the mountain for me?" You are awestruck and feel honored that God would ask you. Quickly you nod in agreement, place the items in your backpack and off you go. Happily, you continue on your journey. A short while after, you encounter a group of children. They approach you and ask politely if you could help carry some of their packs up the hill since their little legs are getting so tired. Of course! Who can say no to the children?

Further up the road, you meet some of your friends. They just finished boxing care packages and are hoping you could take the food to the top of the mountain to their elderly family members. Surely, you are a good friend after all. A mile later, you are approached by a few members of your cherished faith community. "We are all called to do good; please deliver these supplies to our mission partners." The trail starts becoming quite steep and your pack is so heavy. You continue climbing but each step is harder and harder. The weight becomes overwhelming. Angry, you call out to God, "Why have you given me more than I can carry?" God replies, "I only asked you to bring my things to the top of the mountain."

Please substitute a more suitable word or name that represents your spiritual beliefs if appropriate.

o   What is it that you are carrying in your backpack?

o   What are the things that you need to get rid of to lighten the weight?

o   What "items" are you spiritually called to carry, and what "items" are you lugging to please other people?

10 The Workings of My Mind

Jill Bolte Taylor spent her life researching the brain. As a Harvard neuroscientist, Jill dedicated her career to understanding the complexities that constitute the human brain. One day, however, Jill got an insider's look at the organ. On a winter day in 1996, she woke up to a popped blood vessel in her left lobe. The left side of her brain, associated with logic, reason, analysis, ego, and judgment, was off-line. For a short amount of time, Jill experienced the world exclusively through her right brain. Consequently, she described a quiet mind, free of worries. A mind perceiving interconnectedness with all things.

"I looked at my arm, and I realized I could no longer define the boundaries of where I began and where I ended. What were the atoms and molecules of my arm versus the atoms and molecules of the wall? …

Everything blended together as one," she says. "I felt that I was as big as the universe.

"Based upon my experience with losing my left mind, I whole-heartedly believe that the feeling of deep inner peace is neurological circuitry located in our right brain...My stroke of insight would be, peace is only a thought away, and all we have to do to access it, is silence the voice of our dominating left mind."

(Adapted from Jill Bolte Taylor, My Stroke of Insight: A Brain Scientist's Personal Story.)

Neuroscience: The Workings of the Mind

Due to our evolutionary story, human beings have a brain that is wired for survival, not for mental health. At this point, it may be helpful to clarify the difference between the brain and the mind. The brain is the physical and biological source that gives life to the mental processes administered by the mind. In other words, the brain is similar to the hardware of your personal computer and the mind is comparable to installed software programs.

Is it time for an upgrade? Is your mind running programs that are not particularly useful?

Dr. Dan Siegel, a clinical professor of psychiatry, simplifies the triune brain with a hand model.

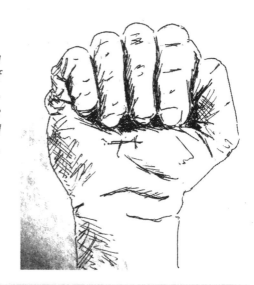

Make a fist, curl the fingers over your thumb. Place both palms touching so the thumbs face upward and look down at your hands. This is a good replica of your two brain halves; your brain is actually about the size of your two connected fists. Most people think that their brain is much larger.

The human brain is organized into three segments. The lowest part, the brain stem, is represented here by the wrist. The brain stem is the most primitive part of the human brain, controlling basic survival functions such as breathing and heart rate. Next, we get to the limbic system, shown here by the thumb. The limbic system is the control center for all things emotion, including urges such as sex, caregiving and power. The hand model concludes with the newest edition to the human brain, the cortex. Humans, by the way, have the largest cerebral cortex compared to other mammals. The Prefrontal Cortex (PFC) is the brain's top executive, managing complex problems through laborious analyses, planning and organization. Characterized here as the fingers curling over the thumb. Make note that the fingers (prefrontal cortex) are touching the thumb (limbic system), indicating linkage between brain structures.

Dr. Siegel speaks about the importance of integration when appreciating a well-functioning brain—not only integration of top brain structures such as the PFC with lower structures such as the limbic system but also integration of both brain halves. Our brain is divided into two distinct hemispheres. The left hemisphere is associated among other tasks with language, linear thinking, analysis and mathematics, whereas the right brain recognizes body language, imagination, intuition, music, art and emotions. Here's how a well-integrated brain includes right and left hemispheres into a decision-making process.

It's time to purchase a new car. The right brain may communicate its desire for a sexy sportscar with a flood of images of you driving a flashy Porsche convertible through the town center, pompously nodding at the pedestrians, whereas your left brain will tell you that a Porsche convertible will not fit all the children you need to pick up for carpool and is not suitable as a family car. Ideally, both brain sides balance each other out and you leave the car dealer with a car that isn't a minivan but is a car that is roomy yet stylish and in vogue.

Who is the Boss?

Thanks to our story of evolution, humans' brains are wired for survival, not mental health. In other words, our brains are far more interested in processing negative information than neutral or positive data. For example, it's nice to stop and take in a beautiful sunset, then again, it does not provide us with an evolutionary advantage. If we, however, focus our attention on this possibly threatening group of people, it may mean life or death. Therefore, our brain is predominantly survival-oriented, concerned with threats, problem-solving and fear-based data processing. Ever wonder why the daily news reports highlight destructive, violent or harmful events? Because our brain habitually turns towards fear-based information in an effort to comprehend the lay of the land and subsequently keep us safe. Who orchestrates this process? A small almond-shaped structure in the brain, the *amygdala*.

Dan Siegel's hand-model provides a visual of an integrated brain. At times, however, our brain can enter a disintegrated brain state, which Dan fondly labels as "flipped your lid." When we flip the lid, we experience a disconnect between the PFC and the limbic region of our brain.

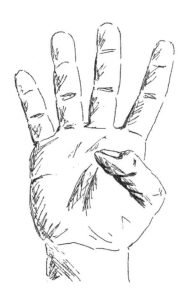

When we lose connection, the Amygdala has activated the fight or flight response; consequently, we experience big emotions such as anger, fear or anxiety. The popular saying "I lost my mind" contains profound physiological truths. The rational and reasonable part of our brain, the PFC, has been taking off-line by the Boss, the amygdala. Everyone's brain is hardwired to allow the amygdala to seize control in times of danger. It turns out that the amygdala's interpretation of what constitutes danger is questionable. We experience fight or flight while being in traffic, working towards a deadline or arguing with a family member. Dangerous situations? Not really. Yet those stimuli cause us to flip our lids.

If you are in a heated argument with your spouse, chances are you are in a dis-integrated brain state, which means that you are physically incapable of fully comprehending what your spouse is trying to communicate. Your state of mind is only interested in you formulating your next line of attack. When this happens, I often instruct clients to THROB.

T – Take a Time out.

H – Halt the interaction, cool off and help your brain re-integrate.

R – Remove yourself from the situation, if possible. Walking or running are great ways to calm down.

O – Observe your thinking. Are your thoughts unhelpful and fueling the emotion?

B – Breath, deep and full breaths. At least 5 deep breaths.

Anxiety can be equated with a hyperactive amygdala, a bit like a smoke detector that goes off anytime someone is in the kitchen cooking. The amygdala is not logical—in fact, it is a highly sensitive brain part that often goes off needlessly.

Rewire the Anxious Brain

The way to retrain the brain is to behave as if there is no threat. Joe, a thirty-year-old car mechanic, started therapy because he became really anxious when initiating conversations with strangers. He wanted to improve on this because of his personal goal of finding a partner. His amygdala interpreted a conversation with a stranger as a threat and initiated the fight or flight process. Joe could feel his heart racing, palms sweating and his face blushing each time he approached someone. So, he would quickly turn around and walk away. Neuroscience tells us that the amygdala can learn not to overreact. The amygdala says, "Prove that you're not scared by behaving without fear and I'll buy it. Until then, my alarm bells are ringing." Joe coached himself to walk up to a person despite feeling nervous. He ignored, as much as possible, the alarm bells. Regardless of his internal turmoil, Joe continued to lean into his fears. Once Joe stopped avoiding these situations, his amygdala learned that nothing bad actually happened when talking with strangers. Each time he walked up to a person, it got easier and easier. The amygdala will adapt if you remain in the situation. When you practice facing your fears, your anxiety will decrease. Avoidance is a like food for the monster: It makes it bigger and stronger.

Positive Neuroplasticity

My family and I love hiking, especially long-distance hikes with a full backpack into remote areas. The close proximity to the Appalachian Trail enables us to do multi-day hikes on the famed AT. Imagine that you are also hiking the AT: You notice how well maintained the pathway is. It's been cleared of trees and a bright white blaze guides the way. It's quite easy to hike along the wide path. What if you decide you'd like a more challenging experience and go off trail?

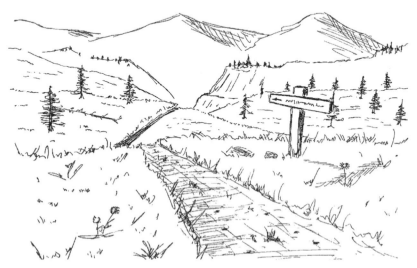

Bushwhacking is extremely difficult due to a multitude of obstacles, from poison ivy to tree roots to thick underbrush. It takes a lot more time to move through the forest and a great deal of effort.

Welcome to the world of neuroplasticity. Neuroplasticity is the ability of the brain to reorganize its patterns of responding. In other words, the brain can create a new pathway, hence the brain is capable of changing your thoughts, feelings and responses. You really can teach an old dog (or brain) new tricks. If you always react to traffic in a highly negative way, you have created a pathway in the brain that makes it more likely that you'll keep reacting to traffic in the same negative way. The promise of neuroplasticity tells you that your brain does not have to react that way if you begin building a new pathway. This new and improved pathway may have you enjoy a favorite podcast while sitting in traffic. You may coach yourself to perceive a traffic jam as an unanticipated gift of time to pray, sing or listen to uplifting music. Each time you remember to use the new pathway, the old one loses momentum. Consequently, you are rewiring the circuitry of your brain.

Practices that help rewire your brain:

- o Face your fears
- o Experience discomfort (what doesn't kill you makes you stronger)
- o Practice gratitude
- o Treat yourself with compassion
- o Tame Amy (*see following chapter practice)
- o Meditate
- o Enjoy silence and solitude
- o Connect with nature
- o Breathe deeply
- o Take breaks
- o Dare to be different, imperfect
- o Seek therapy
- o Be curious about your inner landscape (thoughts, feelings, sensations)

The Power of Metta

Metta, also known as loving-kindness practice, is a form of guided meditation that gently directs the meditator to channel mental energy in two powerful ways. First, you are asked to bring to mind people who love you very much. Imagine these people near you, sending you warm wishes and love. Really bask in the love coming from all the people around you. Visualize overflowing with warmth and love.

Second, you start sending that love and warmth out to others whom you deeply cherish. To help verbalize this notion, the following words can be helpful.

May you experience peace; may you be happy;
may you be free from suffering.

You repeat this phrase silently for two more times. Next, you picture a person whom you don't know very well, someone rather neutral in your life. Just like you, that person wishes to have a good life. So, you send him or her warmth and wishes for happiness.

May your life be filled with happiness, health and
well-being.

Now think of a person whom you have somewhat difficult feelings toward. It could be a relative or a coworker. You and that person share the desire for a happiness.

May you experience peace; may you be happy;
may you be free from suffering.

For some people, this step is challenging, often because the person we envision brings up a lot of intense emotions. Try doing the meditation with someone a bit less upsetting. Or take a step back and stay with visualizing the neutral people. Lastly, you expand your awareness and imagine the whole earth as little ball in front of you, sending warmth and kindness to all living beings.

Just as I wish to, may you live with ease,
happiness and good health.

It's a great deal more effective if you listen to the audio-guided version. There are plenty of resources for you online if you type into your search engine, *"Loving-Kindness guided meditation."* My version is available for download at www.peaceinthewild.com

Why do Metta?

A study done by D. J. Kearney and colleagues in 2013 found that individuals practicing loving-kindness meditation, compared to a control group, had increases in positive emotions, in part due to baseline vagal tone. Vagal tone generally determines parasympathetic nervous system activity, often referred to as the "rest and digest" mode. In other words, Metta practice has a calming effect on our nervous system. Other studies report an increase in gray matter, the home of the brain's neuronal cell bodies, in areas of the brain related to emotion regulation. Increase in grey matter can be understood as positive brain growth.

In summary, these and other studies suggest that loving-kindness meditation increases

- *Love*
- *Joy*
- *Sense of calm*
- *Gratitude*
- *Purpose in life*
- *Life satisfaction*

Therefore, consider integrating this practice into your daily life. Not only you but the people around you will benefit from your commitment.

Practice: Taming Amy(gdala)

Taming Amy is a chart designed to organize a weekly routine to calm the sympathetic nervous system (SNS). Your experience of anxiety is predominantly a physical sensation of the flight or fight response amplifying many systems in your body. Therefore, our first counter-response needs to originate within the body. If we consistently engage in actions that deactivate our SNS, we are rewiring the brain by making Amygdala less likely to fire at the drop of a hat.

Want to take control of your anxiety? Commit to two or three of these practices daily. Most practices suggested here can be found online or through Apps such as Insight Timer, Stop Breath Think, Calm or Simply Being. Here is a brief description of recommended breathing techniques.

o **Alternate Nostril Breathing (PRAMAYAM):** A very effective way to calm the SNS quickly. Easy to learn while watching a YouTube video on Alternate Nostril Breathing.

> 1. The right thumb softly closes the right nostril.
>
> 2. Inhale as slowly as you can through the left nostril.
>
> 3. Next, switch and close the left nostril with your ring finger. Pause. Exhale slowly through the right nostril.
>
> 4. With the right nostril open, inhale slowly.

5. Close the right nostril with the thumb. Pause. Exhale through the left nostril.

6. Inhale through the left. Pause before switching, then close left and exhale through the right.

7. Repeat this pattern five to ten times.

o **Diaphragmatic Breathing:** This type of breathing has you image that your stomach is a balloon that gets pumped up with the inhalation and deflated with the exhalation. Anxiety causes quick and shallow chest breathing to occur which in turn keeps the fight or flight response running. The easiest way to do diaphragmatic breathing is to lay down on your back. Place a small stuffed animal or beanie baby on your navel and give the animal a ride up and down.

o **Full-body breaths:** Imagine that the soles of your feet breath in air, then let the breath travel all the way up your body and out at the top of your head. Notice, even exaggerate, the short pause before the breath enters back into your body, entering at the top of the head, slowly making its way down the body and exiting through the soles of your feet. Continue doing these full body breaths a few more times, following your breathing mentally on its journey through the body.

o **Pursed Lips Out-Breath:** Take a deep, full inbreath. Then pause at the top of your breath before pursing your lips, and as you exhale, allow the breath to create a whooshing sound through the lips as it leaves your body. Inhale—smell the roses. Exhale—blow out the candles.

o **4-7-8 Breath:** As you inhale count to four, and once you have arrived at the top of your breath, pause for a count of seven. Then exhaling slowly and deeply while silently counting to eight. Also, as you exhale, allow your breath to create a whooshing sound through the mouth as it leaves your body. Again, breathe in to a count of four, hold the breath for seven, then release the breath through the mouth while making a whooshing sound until you have reached a count of eight.

11 Ideal Conditions for Mastering the Mind

A belligerent samurai, an old Japanese tale goes, tired of Warcraft, decided one day to go in search of wisdom. He was directed to seek out a wise Zen master who lived on the top of a steep mountain. When he found the monk, the samurai asked permission to enter. He then challenged the Zen master to explain the concept of heaven and hell. But the monk replied with scorn, "You're nothing but a lout—I can't waste my time with the likes of you!"

His very honor attacked, the samurai flew into a rage. Nobody would disrespect him like this. The more he thought about this insolence, the more his anger flared. Finally, pulling his sword from its scabbard, he yelled, "I should kill you for your impertinence."

"That," the monk calmly replied, "is hell."

Startled at seeing the truth in what the master pointed out about the fury that had him in its grip, the samurai calmed down, sheathed his sword, bowed, and asked for forgiveness, then thanked the monk for the insight.

"And that," said the monk, "is heaven."

Ideal Conditions for Mastering the Mind

At times, I speak at employee leadership seminars on organizational effectiveness. Businesses care about profits. Therefore, productivity and effectiveness are priorities in corporations. However, productivity is not always about hammering away at problems. To be productive, we have to put ourselves under the right conditions. Stanford researcher Dr. Ophir suggests that multitasking is less productive than uni-tasking. Mindfulness, for example, resets our brains and temporarily frees us from the emotions that impede decision-making. As we revolutionize our relationship with our mind, we should consider what entails ideal conditions.

Uni-tasking

Why not multi-tasking?

o The brain can only focus on one thing at a time. We take in information sequentially. When we try to focus on multiple tasks simultaneously, what happens is that we switch back and forth between tasks, paying less attention to either task.

o We can chew gum and walk at the same time, but we can't focus on two input-rich activities that require our attention such as composing an email while being on a call.

o It takes on average 50% longer to accomplish a task when we get interrupted, and we are likely to make 50% more errors. That's because when you switch tasks, your brain has to run through a complex process of deactivating certain neurons all the while initiating other neurons.

o Multitasking, busily switching from one task to another, has been shown to activate the reward circuitry in the brain, releasing dopamine. In other words, it can feel good but can add an enormous amount of stress on our system.

o Multitasking can give the illusion of productivity, but it really slows down our processing ability.

Brain Breaks

Consistent breaks for the brain will enable your mind to ward off burn-out and remain clear and uncluttered. Brain break ideas include

o   Three-minute breathing space (simply take three to five minutes to breathe mindfully).

o   Come to your senses. Take a moment to focus on all your senses. What do I feel, hear, see, taste or smell right now?

o   During your lunch break, go outside and take in some fresh air.

o   Listen to a guided meditation a few times per day.

Nature

Habitually engage with nature. Being in a forest or park setting has an incredibly powerful effect on our bodies and brains. Science is proving what we've always known intuitively: Nature does good things to the human brain. Some researchers believe that being in nature allows the prefrontal cortex, the brain's executive command, to decelerate and rest this overworked body part. Stephen and Rachel Kaplan at the University of Michigan speak of attention restoration theory. They argue that the visual elements in natural environments—sunsets, streams, butterflies—reduce stress and mental fatigue. Thus, spending time in natural environments, promotes brain health in addition to a calmer nervous system.

Decrease Negative Self-Talk and Judgment

The mind can easily exaggerate the severity of errors, failures or stumbling blocks. Each time we stand up against the habit of self-critique, whether it's offering ourselves compassion when we are experiencing a challenging mood or reacting reassuringly to a decision we made, we weaken the grip of our conditioning. This mental attitude gives you the wherewithal to pause, observe, and note internal judgement. Then consequently, shift the internal dialog to one of kindness and gentleness. Your mind learns better in an environment of positive regard.

Acceptance/Adaptability vs. Change and Control

Am I under the illusion of having control? What can I really control? Not much. Another reason many people experience anxiety is the false belief that one should have greater control over colleagues, bosses, clients, children, a spouse or traffic.

Notice the stiffest tree is most easily cracked,
while the bamboo or willow survives by bending
with the wind. Chinese Proverb

The mind has a natural resistance to change. The "unknown" activates our flight or fight system. Survival is no longer certain because we can't control what we don't know. The antidote to control is acceptance, as the famous serenity prayer advises us.

God, give me grace to accept with serenity the things that cannot be changed, Courage to change the things which could be changed, and the Wisdom to distinguish the one from the other.

What is the antidote to our mind's natural resistance to change? Reflect on each fear and write down what you would do if that fear came to pass. Knowing you have a back-up plan can really help to defuse emotional apprehension.

Sleep and Food

You already know how important a good night's sleep and healthy food is to your mental health. The National Heart, Lung and Blood Institute recommends 7-8 hours of sleep for adults, yet we often don't get enough sleep as screens engross our minds way past our bedtimes. Lack of enough sleep is linked to "brain-fog." Inadequate sleep creates a feedback loop with depression and anxiety. Here are a couple of guidelines to orient your lifestyle towards better sleep.

Sleep

o *Bedrooms should be used ONLY for sleep and sex.*

o *Be consistent with sleep and wake-up times—the mind likes regularity.*

o *Avoid alcohol, large meals, caffeine, electronics and the news at least two hours before bedtime.*

The food one eats influences the neurotransmitters or chemical messengers of the brain. In turn, neurotransmitters affect our moods. Furthermore, the brain influences the gut-stress relationship. Inflammation is linked with depression and anxiety. Healthy gut bacteria shapes behavior as well as emotional responses. In other words, we can improve our mental health with the food we eat.

Daily Eating for Improved Mood

o *Three meals per day, snacks if needed*

o *Lean protein, unsaturated fats, complex carbs, lots of colorful vegetables*

o *Minimize processed and packaged food*

o *Include prebiotic and probiotic*

o *Avoid caffeine, alcohol and tobacco*

Shopping List for Improved Mood

- Eggs
- Fish
- Fruit
- Avocado
- Wheatgerm
- Low-fat cheese
- Lean poultry
- Green leafy vegetables
- Seeds
- Nuts

For more information on the topic of mental health and nutrition, explore Dr. Emeran Mayer's book, The Mind-Gut Connection: How the Hidden Conversation Within Our Bodies Impacts Our Mood, Our Choices, and Our Overall Health.

Positive Neuroplasticity

Rick Hanson, a psychologist affiliated with UC Berkeley, has spent many years researching happiness. He believes we can rewire our brains to become more resilient and consequently experience deeper happiness. Every time you have a thought, your brain cells fire and wire a certain way.

With enough repetition, we get good at hitting a tennis ball, and with enough repetition, we get good at thinking a certain way.

Let's say that whenever I think of my mother-in-law, my mind pulls up negatively-charged memories, and the process becomes stronger each time. Once I disengage from this autopilot and direct my attention on a different memory or thought-pattern, I am practicing self-directed neuroplasticity. It's me taking control. Positive neuroplasticity is the brain's ability to rewire itself to create a more upbeat state of mind. But this takes intention and effort.

Hanson urges us to exercise a technique he calls "Taking in the Good." He believes that just three simple steps can reduce our mind's negativity bias and boost happiness:

Seek. Savor. Soak.

o **Step 1:** Seek for positive details in your life. Transform them into experiences.

o **Step 2:** Savor the positive experience by dwelling on it for at least 30 seconds. Feel it in the   body.   Notice the emotions. Magnify the experience.

o **Step 3:** Soak it in. Have the intention to let the experience soak into your body and mind.

For example, I enjoy a cup of breakfast tea in the morning. I never really thought about it much, but I am grateful for this little A.M. pleasure. Ordinarily, I'd drink my tea while reading the latest news updates on my smartphone. When "Taking in the Good," my tea experience looks a little different.

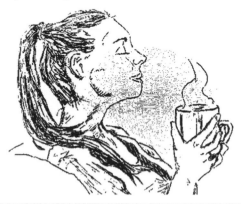

o **Step 1:** English breakfast tea in the morning is a positive occurrence in my life. I put my phone away and stand by the window looking out at the morning mist. I experience my tea as the multiple flavors warm my tongue. I detect a hint of sugar and milk. I sense the tea on my tongue and as it warms my body.

o **Step 2:** I remind myself to savor this experience and stay with the flavors, the warmth, the smell, the view of my yard for a good minute or so. I notice that my body is warming up. I feel content.

o **Step 3:** This experience is good. Even though my mind wants to rush to the next thing, I remain in the moment. I tell myself to soak it in. I imagine that this experience emits a soft warm glow that enters my body which in turn sends the warm light out. I have now rewired my brain toward positivity.

Taking in the Good is similar to practicing gratitude. The two practices are connected. Perhaps gratitude is a natural precursor to Taking in the Good as we first recall positive things in our lives. Gratitude doesn't have to be limited to the big three: health, family, and work. It's the small things that truly bring joy into our lives. Walking the dog, the smell of coffee, chocolate, clothes that fit, a sunny day, the first snowfall, flowers, cuddling with our loved-one, a funny movie, a reliable car, a comfy bed. Returning from a camping trip helps me remember all the comforts of my home that I am so grateful for, especially a hot shower.

A colleague of mine once told me a story about a client who was deeply depressed and suicidal. He had been struggling for years and finally came to the conclusion that it was simply too painful to continue living. He granted himself permission to end his life. The only thing that diminished his resolve was the love for his daughter. He concluded that he would give himself one more year, and if in 365 days he did not sense any improvement, he would commit suicide. He understood that expecting a different result without making any changes was the definition of insanity; he pledged to make a simple life change. He would note down, every evening, a list of things that he was grateful for. No matter how dark the day was, he had to come up with at least three things. At first the practice felt artificial and futile. With time, however, a mental shift occurred. He reported spending less mental energy on what was wrong with his life and more time on good occurrences. Needless to say, he did not commit suicide as his emotional pain slowly diminished.

Your Mindful Evolution

Mindfulness, or the ability to stay present with acceptance, can be seen as a personal evolution. The capability to anchor in the present moment will develop and progress over time. Depending on your stage in life, you may or may not have the time and resources to dedicate to the practice of present-moment-awareness. The following chart parallels human developmental stages with mindfulness strategies. Children, for example, approach mindfulness quite differently than adults.

Infant

Dependent on the caregiver. Building attachment bonds with caregivers. This is the precursor for healthy attachment in future relationships.

Infants need caregivers to be present with them. Mindfulness can begin when caregivers avoid distractions and are present with the baby. Making eye contact and mirroring smiles are ways to introduce mindfulness. Walking meditation while cuddling the baby can be especially calming to both parent and child.

Toddler

Discovering the world and its limits.

Create a family lifestyle of mindfulness. Hands-on activities to help anchor in the present moment. "What does this clay feel like?" "Let's roll the clay into a ball and roll it over in our hands." "Let's blow on the pinwheel and see if we can't notice our breath." Mindfulness practice can also help mom and dad surf the wave of a tantrum instead of getting swept up by negative emotions.

School Age

Learning new things, exploring creativity and forming social connections.

Children at this age are inherently mindful. They are curious and awe-struck quite naturally. Encourage them to use their five "Spidey-Senses" to home in on the present moment. Use nature as an ally. Discovery walks in nature encourage children to describe all the things they hear, smell or see as if for the first time.

Adolescent

Intense physical changes, emotional drive for independence, focus on peer relationships.

Being an adolescent can be stressful. At times, this age can bring up peer pressure and test one's self-confidence. Help teens understand the role of the mind in creating unhelpful thoughts. Numerous meditation apps can support a teenager in integrating deep-breathing and mindfulness into their day. Perhaps experimenting with a social-media fast would be intriguing.

Young Adulthood

Transition to independence. Establishing oneself in the world. Familiarizing oneself with the responsibilities of becoming an adult. Attention to romantic relationships and commitment.

As life becomes more demanding and responsibilities start adding up, mindfulness practice becomes ever more urgent. Incorporating short mindfulness exercises into the workday can be a real antidote to stress. Smartphone reminders can help us remember this commitment. Other techniques include a one-minute meditation on one's body, thoughts or emotions. Single-tasking, when possible, helps reduce cognitive overload. A ten-minute outdoor walk at lunch time can reboot the mind. Limiting time on devices is necessary. The pinging of a text or email can wreak havoc on concentration and effectiveness.

Middle Adulthood

Child rearing and home making takes precedence. Emphasis on career development and enterprise.

At this stage in life, people are often hard-working and extremely busy. One must find clever ways to create mindful moments. Any chore can be done mindfully. If it's cooking, doing the dishes or commuting to work, one can rest the attention on the task at hand. The sound of plates, the smell of the dish detergent, the feel of the water on the hand. Training the mind to stay in the here and now and not check off the mental to-do list.

Late Adulthood

Retirement often leads to motivation to give back to one's community or get involved in the lives of grandchildren.

Health problems can increase at this stage. Mindfulness practice can be helpful as it can shift the mind's attention away from what's wrong to what is right in one's life. Mindful awareness can give rise to connectedness and meaning-making which in turn is linked to well-being. A nature visualization, such as placing thoughts onto leaves and watching them drift downstream, can aid in releasing anxious beliefs.

Death and Dying

Terminal illness, hospice, death and dying.

"When the time comes to go, when the doctors have to throw up their hands in helplessness, the skill you have been developing in your meditation is the one thing that won't

abandon you. It will enable you to handle your death with finesse. Even though we don't like to think about it, death is going to come no matter what, so we should learn how to stare it down. Remember that a death well-handled is one of the surest signs of a life well lived."

-Venerable Thanissaro Bhikku

Practice: Gratitude Practice

We think too much about what goes wrong and not enough about what goes right in our lives. Of course, sometimes it makes sense to analyze bad events so that we can learn from them and avoid them in the future. However, people tend to spend more time thinking about the negative than is helpful. Worse, this focus on undesirable events sets us up for anxiety and depression. One way to keep this from happening is to get better at contemplating and savoring what went well.

Daily Gratitude Practice:

- Write down three things that went well today. You may use a journal or your computer to record the events, but it is important that you have a physical record of what you wrote. The three things need not be earthshattering in importance ("My husband picked up my favorite ice cream for dessert on the way home from work today"), but they can be important ("My sister just gave birth to a healthy baby boy").

- Next to each positive event, answer the question "Why did this happen?" For example, if you wrote that your husband picked up ice cream, write "because my husband is really thoughtful sometimes" or "because I remembered to call him from work and remind him to stop by the grocery store." Or if you wrote, "My sister just gave birth to a healthy baby boy," you might pick as the cause "She engaged in healthy lifestyle during her pregnancy."

Writing about why the positive events in your life happen may seem awkward at first, but please stick with it for one week. It will get easier.

Dr. Martin Seligman, expert scholar of positive psychology, promises that individuals will be "less depressed, happier, and addicted to this exercise six months from now."

12

My Life Compass

A water bearer in India had two large pots; each hung on an end of a pole which he carried across his neck. One of the pots had a crack in it, and while the other pot was perfect and always delivered a full portion of water at the end of the long walk from the stream to the master's house, the cracked pot arrived only half full. For a full two years this went on daily, with the bearer delivering only one-and-a-half pots full of water in his master's house. Of course, the perfect pot was proud of its accomplishments, perfect to the end for which it was made. But the poor cracked pot was ashamed of its own imperfection, and miserable that it was able to accomplish only half of what it had been made to do. After two years of what it perceived to be a bitter failure, it spoke to the water bearer one day by the stream.

"I am ashamed of myself, and I want to apologize to you."

"Why?" asked the bearer. "What are you ashamed of?"

"I have been able, for these past two years, to deliver only half my load because this crack in my side causes water to leak out all the way back to your master's house. Because of my flaws, you have to do all of this work, and you don't get full value from your efforts," the pot said.

The water bearer felt sorry for the old cracked pot, and in his compassion, he said, "As we return to the master's house, I want you to notice the beautiful flowers along the path." Indeed, as they went up the hill, the old cracked pot took notice of the sun warming the beautiful wildflowers on the side of the path, and this cheered it some. But at the end of the trail, it still felt bad because it had leaked out half its load, and so again the pot apologized to the bearer for its failure.

The bearer said to the pot, "Did you notice that there were flowers only on your side of your path, but not on the other side? That's because I have always known about your flaw, and I took advantage of it. I planted flower seeds on your side of the path, and every day while we walk back from the stream, you've watered them. For two years I have been able to pick these beautiful flowers to decorate my master's table. Without you being just the way, you are, he would not have this beauty to grace his house."

Letting Go of Imperfection

I love this story because it so beautifully illustrates how "imperfections" can be a positive force in the world. I know for a fact that my own struggle with anxiety has helped me empathize and comprehend my clients' struggles on a deeper level. How would our life change if we could make peace with our shortcomings and accept ourselves as we are?

Often, I witness people waging war against themselves as they reject their body and their mind, daily. Cheryl Strayed tells a story of acceptance in her memoir Wild. Cheryl wages war on herself in the aftermath of her mother's death. The most profound moment of her recovery comes as she radically accepts her past destructive decisions. "What if I had no regrets?" "What if all the horrible things that I did guided me to this exact moment?" A heartfelt gesture of reconciliation with oneself.

Perfectionism is a particularly potent fuel for anxiety. Perfection punishes failure and consequently powers self-loathing. Imagine you are a student who has a teacher who habitually reprimands you for inaccuracies or errors: How would you feel about learning in his or her classroom? And yet that is exactly what happens when we demand perfection without grace. How would our relationship with ourselves change if we rewarded progress not perfection? I once heard the analogy of a hammer. A hammer has the energy to build or to destroy. Can we allow our imperfections to build us up instead of being a force of destruction?

Creating a Life Compass

My 12-year-old son had just earned his scouting orienteering merit badge a few months before we ventured on our family vacation to Yosemite. After receiving our wilderness permit, we hit the trail for the backcountry. The beauty of the landscape was overwhelming, and the June sun was warming our backs. Our trek along a rugged mountain path was clearly marked and easy to follow. A few hours into the hike we encountered snow. As we continued hiking, the snow began covering the trail. At some point, the snow was so deep that all signs of a footpath had disappeared. This was the moment for my son, Sebastian, to shine. He smugly pulled out his compass and said, "Let me take it from here." Pinning his compass next to our detailed trail map, he calculated our whereabouts and led the way. I swear he grew several inches taller when we arrived back at our car four days later.

A compass helps us clarify where we are and what directions we want to head. It's been my experience that when we struggle with fear and anxiety, we lose our sense of direction. We only receive guidance from our fears. Our fears have covered the trail we want to hike.

A person's life compass is guided by values. Damian had found love again at age 65. After a long, toxic divorce, he could not believe his luck to finally be in a relationship with a woman who valued a similar lifestyle and hobbies. They shared a love for travel. Damian valued Tina's sense of adventure and independent spirit. A few months into the relationship, Damian noticed worries creeping into his thoughts.

"Why is she spending so much time traveling with friends, when she could be with me? What if this relationship doesn't work out, then I will feel so lonely. I can't believe she is spending money on a scuba diving course when I don't like scuba diving; she must not really care about me."

As Damian spent more and more time entertaining these anxious thoughts, the more isolated he felt. Damian was being led astray by his fears. His values and fears were an opposing force, creating internal turmoil. I asked him once if his thoughts moved him closer to or farther away from his values. He recognized then that he had lost his way.

Live life consciously and consistently with what you value. Do so mindfully and with compassion. Then your life and everything you want to be about will come into focus.

Values and the Shining Lighthouse

Living on the east coast of the United States, I have developed an affinity for lighthouses. They come in many different shapes and sizes but are united in their mission to provide a guiding light to small and large craft navigating the ocean waters. Values are the shining lighthouse in the sea of life, orienting you in the direction you want to go. Envision each brick of the lighthouse as representing one of your values. The foundation is now laid. There is room for renovations as we grow older; values may change. The beacon is sent out to call you back home. "Come this way: This is what you're are all about."

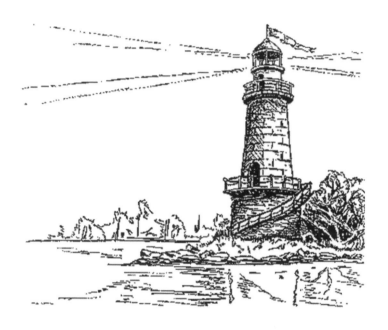

Frequently, I observe incongruency between a client's values and their current lifestyle. It's been my experience that the larger the incongruency is, the more pronounced their mental health challenges. Once you become clear what the bricks of your lighthouse consist of, reflect on how accurate your present-day life reflects those values. For example, if one of your top values is being a lifelong learner but you are not engaging in any form of studying, you are not actively fostering the ideals you believe in.

Victor Frankl's Logotherapy

Growing up in Germany left me with an intimate understanding of a very dark time in history: the rise of Nazi Germany and the consequent Holocaust. It's difficult to describe the generational trauma still haunting the people of Germany. Being connected to the perpetrators of one of the evilest human atrocities in history leaves its mark even centuries later. Reading Frankl's *Man's Search for Meaning* in college was a surprisingly emotional encounter for me. Frankl's description of his life in a concentration camp and subsequent insights launched a therapeutic approach know as logotherapy. In essence, Frankl observed that a prisoner's ability to create meaning would be a determining element of their ability to survive. Frankl believed that if there is meaning in life, there must also be meaning in suffering.

"When a man finds that it is his destiny to suffer, he will have to accept his suffering as his task; his single and unique task. He will have to acknowledge that fact that even in suffering he is unique and alone in the universe. No one can relieve him of his suffering or suffer in his place. His unique opportunity lies in the way in which he bears his burden... As we said before, any attempt to restore a man's inner strength in the camp had first to succeed in showing him some future goal. Recall the renown philosopher Nietzsche's words, 'he who has a '*why*' to live for can bear with almost any '*how*.'"

Therefore, logotherapy is based on the notion that "striving to find meaning in one's life is the primary motivational force in man" (Frankl, 1984, p 121).

According to logotherapy, meaning in life can be found in three ways:

o   Through work or deed

o   By experiencing someone or something

o   Our attitude toward suffering

At any giving moment in time, life asks to answer its call. Purpose and meaning are the life forces that propel us forward.

o   What is your purpose in life at this moment in time?

o   What were some of the most meaningful moments of your life?

o   When have you felt most deeply and fully alive?

o   What legacy do you want to leave behind?

o   Name three relationships that are meaningful to you?

o   Do you find your work to be meaningful?

o   Can you reflect on a difficulty in your life and find a possible purpose for this struggle?

Practice: My Values and Life Mission

My Values and Mission: A Reflective Exercise

Goal: Systematically gain clarity of what you value most in life.

1. Conduct a value-card sort. This usually comprises sorting through a deck of cards. Each card describes something that may represent a personal value for you. Look at each card and decide if it describes a value you hold dearly. The goal is to narrow the deck in a way that you have no more than 10 cards at the end.

2. Now I'd like you to focus on the values you chose and sort them from 1 to 10. In spot #1 you will put the card that is your top value. Then put your second top value at #2 and so on.

3. Finally, you will try to compose a draft mission statement for your life. Make sure that your top values inform this process. See sample mission

statements as a starting point. Possibly, a life verse from a sacred religious text is part of your mission statement.

Sample Mission Statements

- My purpose for being on this earth is to help others recognize, develop, and use their God-given intuitive abilities to ease suffering and grow in goodness, love, compassion, and wisdom. My desire is to help each of us connect to the love that is eternal—that is the reason for our existence.

- My mission is to be happy and to be part of making other people happy as well. I will do this by working continuously with my personal development from my basic values and virtues.

- I will look for strengths in others and the good in every situation. I will ensure that I do what I can to create a learning environment everywhere I go. I will live with an attitude of gratitude. I will repay every kindness shown to me. I will live, work, and play with renewed spirit.

> **Tip:** Enter into your search engine value card sort. You'll find several online links to PDF files with value card decks.

Practice: Listening to My Values Instead

Often, we simply agree with whatever the mind produces, without any critical analysis if the thought is actually telling the truth. Consequently, we walk down the wrong path. It's crucial that we investigate thought processes with introspection and diligence. This chart illustrates how the mind can fabricate thoughts that oppose our value system. Find examples from your own life.

What my negative thoughts tell me:	I have too much to do. If I don't get everything done, I have failed.
When I listen to the thoughts	I feel overwhelmed.
What my values tell me:	I value progress over perfection. I value self-care.
When I listen to my values:	I feel good about the progress I have made.
Choose what to listen to	If I listen to my thoughts, I do nothing. If I listen to my values. I'll do the best I can—not more.

Final Thoughts

The American Tourist and Mexican Fisherman

An American tourist was at the pier of a small coastal Mexican village when a small boat with just one fisherman docked.

Inside the small boat were several large yellowfin tuna. The tourist complimented the Mexican on the quality of his fish and asked how long it took to catch them.

The Mexican replied, "Only a little while."

The tourist then asked, "Why didn't you stay out longer and catch more fish?"

The Mexican said, "With this I have more than enough to support my family's needs."

The tourist then asked, "But what do you do with the rest of your time?"

The Mexican fisherman said, "I sleep late, fish a little, play with my children, take siesta with my wife, Maria, stroll into the village each evening where I sip wine and play guitar with my amigos. I have a full and busy life."

The tourist scoffed, "I can help you. You should spend more time fishing, and with the proceeds, buy a bigger boat. With the proceeds from the bigger boat you could buy several boats. Eventually you would have a fleet of fishing boats. Instead of selling your catch to a middleman you would sell directly to the processor, eventually opening your own cannery. You would control the product, processing and distribution. You could leave this small coastal fishing village and move to Mexico City, then Los Angeles and eventually New York where you could run your ever-expanding enterprise."

The Mexican fisherman asked, "But, how long will this all take?"

The tourist replied, "15 to 20 years."

"But what then?" asked the Mexican.

The tourist laughed and said, "That's the best part. When the time is right, you would sell your company stock to the public and become very rich; you would make millions."

"Millions? Then what?"

The American said, "Then you would retire. Move to a small coastal fishing village where you would sleep late, fish a little, play with your kids, take siesta with your wife, stroll

185

to the village in the evenings where you could sip wine and play your guitar with your amigos."

My clients often embark on their therapeutic journey with the desire for greater happiness. "When my anxiety is gone, then I will be truly happy. "When I get that better-paying job, then I will be truly happy." "When I find my true love, then I will finally be happy." My personal version of this mirage sounded like this: "When I get my doctorate research completed, then I will be happy." Then it merged into "When I graduate with my PhD, then I will be completely at peace with myself and happy." One of the most difficult realizations was that those three letters after my name did not magically generate peace and contentment after all. The disappointment was intense. Perhaps I just needed to author a book and then that elusive sense of happiness would surely arrive. Looking back, I recognize the foolishness of those thought processes.

All of us struggle on some level with feeling "less than." So, we march on in search of the one person or thing that will banish our sense of inferiority. The life lesson is that there is absolutely nothing external that can create lasting well-being and happiness. Happiness is an internal experience of gratitude for our deep connection to all things. Hopefully, you have begun integrating the practices of this book into your life and have discovered a path leading out of anxiety-land into an experience of joy and inner peace.

References

Introduction

Kabat-Zinn, Jon. *Wherever you go, there you are: Mindfulness meditation in everyday life*. Hachette Books, 2009.

Chapter 2

Chodron, Pema. *When Things Fall Apart: Heart Advice for Difficult Times*. Shambhala Publications, 2000.

Chapter 4

Goleman, Daniel. *Emotional Intelligence*. Bantam, 1996.

O'Grady, K. A., Rollison, D. G., Hanna, T. S., Schreiber-Pan, H., & Ruiz, M. A. (2012). Earthquake in Haiti: Relationship with the Sacred in Times of Trauma. *Journal of Psychology and Theology* 40: 289-301.

Tedeschi, Richard G., and Lawrence G. Calhoun. (1996). The Posttraumatic Growth Inventory: Measuring the Positive Legacy of Trauma. *Journal of Traumatic Stress* 9: 455-471.

Chapter 5

Kondo, Marie, and Emily Woo Zeller. *The Life-changing Magic of Tidying Up*. Findaway World LLC, 2015.

Chapter 6

Hanh Nhat, Thich. *The Art of Power*. HarperOne, 2007.

Chapter 8

Borgonovi, F. (2008). Doing Well by Doing Good. The Relationship Between Formal Volunteering and Self-reported Health and Happiness. *Social Science & Medicine* 66: 232-233.

Neff, Kristin D., Kristin L. Kirkpatrick, and Stephanie S. Rude. (2007). Self-compassion and Adaptive Psychological Functioning. *Journal of Research in Personality* 41: 139-154.

Palmer, Parker J. *Let Your Life Speak: Listening for the Voice of Vocation*. John Wiley & Sons, 1999.

Chapter 9

Cloud, Dr. Henry, and Dr. John Townsend, Boundaries: *When to Say Yes, When to Say No, to Take Control of Your Life*. Zondervan Publishing House, 1992.

Chapter 10

Kearney, David J., et al. (2013). Loving-kindness Meditation for Posttraumatic Stress Disorder: A pilot Study. *Journal of Traumatic Stress* 26: 426-434.

Taylor, Jill Bolte. *My Stroke of Insight*. Hachette UK, 2009.

Siegel, Daniel J. Mindsight: *The New Science of Personal Transformation*. Bantam, 2010.

Chapter 11

Ophir, Eyal, Clifford Nass, and Anthony D. Wagner. (2009). Cognitive Control in Media Multitaskers. *Proceedings of the National Academy of Sciences* 106: 15583-15587.

Seligman, Martin, and Mihaly Csikszentmihalyi. *Positive Psychology: An Introduction*. American Psychological Association, 2000.

Kaplan, Rachel, and Stephen Kaplan. *The Experience of Nature: A Psychological Perspective*. CUP Archive, 1989.

National Heart, Lung, and Blood Institute. *Your Guide to Healthy Sleep*. NIH Publication, 2006.

Mayer, Emeran A. Gut feelings: The Emerging Biology of Gut–brain Communication. (2011). *Nature Reviews Neuroscience* 12: 453.

Hanson, Rick. *Positive Neuroplasticity: The Neuroscience of Mindfulness*. In Advances in Contemplative Psychotherapy, pp. 48-60. Routledge, 2017.

Chapter 12

Frankl, Viktor E. *Man's Search for Meaning*. Simon and Schuster, 1985.

Strayed, Cheryl. *Wild: From Lost to Found on the Pacific Crest Trail*. Vintage, 2012.

About the Author

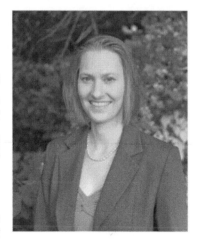

Heidi Schreiber-Pan, Ph.D., is a successful psychotherapist, clinical director and sought-after speaker on topics of resilience, anxiety, neuroscience, and occupational burnout.

Heidi lives with her husband, two teenage boys and her loveable dog Koda, in Baltimore County.

For more information on the author, please go to www.heidischreiberpan.com

Made in the USA
Middletown, DE
16 September 2022

10600600R00113